Temporomandibular Disorders

A Problem-Based Approach

T0176962

Dedication

This edition is dedicated to the memory of Robin Gray. You left finger-prints of grace on my academic career path. You shan't be forgotten.

For my 2Ms: my wife Manal and son-in-law Mohsi

For my 3Ls: Loujin, Lilas, and Leanne

Temporomandibular Disorders

A Problem-Based Approach

Second Edition

Dr M. Ziad Al-Ani
BDS, Oral Surg PG Dip, Fixed Pros PG Dip, MSc, PhD, MFDS RCS(Ed), FHEA
Senior Lecturer
Glasgow Dental Hospital and School
University of Glasgow
Glasgow, UK

Dr Robin J.M. Gray
(1951 – 2019)
BDS, MDS, PhD, MFGDP RCS(Eng), FFDS RCS(Ed), FHEA
Specialist in Oral Surgery
Formerly Director of Manchester Dental Specialists
Formerly Senior Lecturer, Coordinator of TMD Clinical Teaching and Research Services, Department of Dental Medicine and Surgery, University Dental Hospital of Manchester, Manchester, UK
Formerly Principal of Grays Dental Care, General Dental Practice

WILEY Blackwell

Registered Offices
John Wiley & Sons, Inc., 111 River Street, Hoboken, NJ 07030, USA
John Wiley & Sons Ltd, The Atrium, Southern Gate, Chichester, West Sussex, PO19 8SQ, UK

Editorial Office
9600 Garsington Road, Oxford, OX4 2DQ, UK

For details of our global editorial offices, customer services, and more information about Wiley products visit us at www.wiley.com.

Wiley also publishes its books in a variety of electronic formats and by print-on-demand. Some content that appears in standard print versions of this book may not be available in other formats.

Limit of Liability/Disclaimer of Warranty
The contents of this work are intended to further general scientific research, understanding, and discussion only and are not intended and should not be relied upon as recommending or promoting scientific method, diagnosis, or treatment by physicians for any particular patient. In view of ongoing research, equipment modifications, changes in governmental regulations, and the constant flow of information relating to the use of medicines, equipment, and devices, the reader is urged to review and evaluate the information provided in the package insert or instructions for each medicine, equipment, or device for, among other things, any changes in the instructions or indication of usage and for added warnings and precautions. While the publisher and authors have used their best efforts in preparing this work, they make no representations or warranties with respect to the accuracy or completeness of the contents of this work and specifically disclaim all warranties, including without limitation any implied warranties of merchantability or fitness for a particular purpose. No warranty may be created or extended by sales representatives, written sales materials or promotional statements for this work. The fact that an organization, website, or product is referred to in this work as a citation and/or potential source of further information does not mean that the publisher and authors endorse the information or services the organization, website, or product may provide or recommendations it may make. This work is sold with the understanding that the publisher is not engaged in rendering professional services. The advice and strategies contained herein may not be suitable for your situation. You should consult with a specialist where appropriate. Further, readers should be aware that websites listed in this work may have changed or disappeared between when this work was written and when it is read. Neither the publisher nor authors shall be liable for any loss of profit or any other commercial damages, including but not limited to special, incidental, consequential, or other damages.

Library of Congress Cataloging-in-Publication Data

Names: Gray, Robin J. M., author. | Al-Ani, M. Ziad, author.
Title: Temporomandibular disorders : a problem-based approach / Dr. M. Ziad
    Al-Ani, Dr. Robin J.M. Gray.
Description: Second edition. | Hoboken, NJ : Wiley-Blackwell, 2021. | Robin
    J.M. Gray's name appears first in the previous edition. | Includes
    bibliographical references and index.
Identifiers: LCCN 2020053090 (print) | LCCN 2020053091 (ebook) | ISBN
    9781119618744 (paperback) | ISBN 9781119618768 (adobe pdf) | ISBN
    9781119618751 (epub)
Subjects: MESH: Temporomandibular Joint Disorders–therapy |
    Temporomandibular Joint Disorders–diagnosis | Temporomandibular
    Joint–physiopathology
Classification: LCC RK470 (print) | LCC RK470 (ebook) | NLM WU 140.5 |
    DDC 617.5/22–dc23
LC record available at https://lccn.loc.gov/2020053090
LC ebook record available at https://lccn.loc.gov/2020053091

Cover Design: Wiley
Cover Image: © agsandrew/iStock/Getty Images

Set in 10/12.5pt SabonLTStd by SPi Global, Chennai, India
Printed in Singapore

M100906_010321

Contents

Preface to the Second Edition

This is the second edition of *Temporomandibular Disorders: A problem-based approach*. This edition is an updated and revised copy of the first edition to enhance making clinical relevance immediately accessible to the reader.

All chapters have been revisited and two new chapters were added. More colour photographs have been used and flowcharts have been added in Appendix I for a brief description of some essential concepts in this field. A link in the text was added with a symbol indicating the number of the relevant flowcharts at the end. The text has been updated with many new relevant sections. There are two new chapters on evidence-based splint therapy management as well as the aetiology and management of bruxism. These are evolving and dynamic topics which need continuous updating. Some chapters have changed relatively little, such as Orofacial pain and You and the Lawyer, but the importance of these two aspects have been highlighted in different sections of the book. Self-directed learning is critical to develop understanding and some new questions were added to Appendix III. References have been updated and the most relevant evidence-based references and other key papers were included in the Further Reading of each chapter.

This edition, sadly, did not witness the contribution of Robin Gray. He died shortly after the book proposal of this second edition was submitted.

This book sets out to establish some new concepts and philosophies in temporomandibular disorder (TMD) learning. It contains a series of everyday situations that will be encountered in practice. The answers are there but it is up to the reader to find them!

Learning is a dynamic process and those who are involved actively will gain more than passive recipients of knowledge. Problem- or enquiry-based learning should provoke thought and arouse readers' curiosity, motivating them to learn and guiding them into creative thinking. Giving readers a real-life clinical scenario will structure their thoughts, increasing the effectiveness of information delivery and lead to a logical conclusion.

The case histories are stand alone, and each should contain sufficient information for the reader to reach the correct diagnosis and formulate a correct treatment plan that is in the patient's best interests.

There will inevitably be some repetition in the text especially in relation to the chapters on anatomy, function, pathology, classification, and clinical examination. This is because we did not want the reader to have to constantly cross-refer to earlier chapters when reading the case histories. Although there will be some duplication, the case histories will introduce new facts of specific relevance to that situation. We hope that this will meet students' demands because the earlier chapters which are for information can be applied in the later case studies.

There is a unique link to an online interactive quiz (www.wiley.com/go/al-ani/temporomandibular-disorders-2e). This quiz aims not only to test your knowledge of TMD but also to make reading this book more enjoyable, stimulating, and productive.

We have provided a further reading list of relevant evidence-based articles which, as far as possible, are either from systematic reviews or randomised controlled trials published in evidence-based dentistry journals. Therefore, they provide the most up-to-date information.

The final chapters are practical guides of how to make splints and samples of patient information sheets that can be used as templates. We hope therefore that we have addressed not only WHY but also HOW.

Acknowledgements

The author wishes to acknowledge the kind permission of the British Dental Journal in reproducing the annotated images, and Dr Paul Rea and Caroline Morris at the University of Glasgow for the anatomy figures annotated in Chapter 2.

Denise Margaret Coogan has been kind in permitting us to use her as a photographic model in Chapters 3 and 17.

I am very grateful to Tanya McMullin and Loan Nguyen for the advice and support in the production of this text.

About the Companion Website

Don't forget to visit the companion website for this book:

www.wiley.com/go/al-ani/temporomandibular-disorders-2e

There you will find valuable material designed to enhance your learning, including multiple choice questions.

Scan this QR code to visit the companion website

Chapter 1

About the Book

About temporomandibular disorders: what is a 'TMD'?

The term 'temporomandibular disorders' (TMD) covers a constellation of conditions. There have been many attempts to categorise these conditions but all have shortfalls. Some classify by anatomy, some by aetiology, and some by frequency of presentation. We should be aware, however, that there is considerable overlap in any classification system because these are often not clinically appropriate. No one system, therefore, satisfies all the criteria.

TMD affect the articulatory system, consisting of the temporomandibular joints, mandibular muscles, and the occlusion.

Any factor that has an effect on one part of the system is likely to influence other parts of the system, so it is important to avoid tunnel vision when considering possible signs and symptoms of a TMD.

As a dentist in practice, you will inevitably encounter patients with symptoms of a TMD, who may present with facial pain, earache, toothache, jaw joint sounds, or limited movement.

It is estimated that between 50% and 70% of the population will at some stage in their life exhibit some sign of a TMD. This may be subclinical and the patient might not relate the signs to a jaw problem.

In about 20%, these signs will develop into symptoms, which implies that the patient will take notice of hitherto ignored signs, and about 5% of the population will seek treatment. This will happen if the symptoms become intrusive in day-to-day life. It is important for you, as a dentist, to identify these patients and recognise their particular needs and treatment requirements.

The patient may attend complaining of toothache because their natural assumption would be that a tooth was causing the problem, but your role as a clinician is to diagnose the actual cause of the symptoms.

Temporomandibular Disorders: A Problem-Based Approach, Second Edition. M. Ziad Al-Ani and Robin J.M. Gray.
© 2021 M. Ziad Al-Ani and Robin J.M. Gray. Published 2021 by John Wiley & Sons Ltd.
Companion Website: www.wiley.com/go/al-ani/temporomandibular-disorders-2e

A patient presenting with a TMD may have symptoms, in any combination, which might include preauricular or facial pain, restriction or alteration of the range of mandibular movement, muscle pain that is worse with function, localised jaw joint pain, jaw joint sounds such as clicking or crepitation, unexplained tooth sensitivity, tooth or restoration fracture, and chronic daily headache. You must be able to diagnose what is and what is not appropriate for you to treat.

All treatment should be evidence-based. Numerous treatments, either on their own or in combination, have been proposed in accordance with various aetiological theories of TMD. A wide range of pharmacological, occlusal alteration, psychotherapeutic, and physiotherapeutic treatments have also been suggested for the management of TMD, mainly aimed at the reduction of pain and improving the range of movement.

This is possibly the area of most contention in TMD management. Several treatments have been proposed which are not evidence- or scientifically based and when the literature is critically evaluated it is obvious they have little rationale. It is not sufficient to argue that if a treatment modality is published in a journal, which may not be subject to peer review, be un-refereed, or is accessible through the Internet, then it is validated. The dentist has a responsibility only to prescribe treatment for patients that has a proven therapeutic value and ignorance of currently accepted views of what a reasonable body of dentists would do is not an excuse.

All TMD managements and treatments discussed in this second edition of the book are based, as much as possible, on scientific evidence and on sound clinical judgment in cases where only partial evidence or contradictory data were found.

About the book

In modern dental schools, there is a shift from traditional teaching to more interactive methods. In classical didactic textbooks, readers are frequently seen as passive recipients of information, without any engagement in the learning process. Problem-based learning increases the effectiveness of delivering information and makes learning a more memorable experience for the reader.

A green flag denotes a positive pathway and suggests that the reader should follow this train of thought.

A red flag signals caution and suggests that the reader should think hard about this aspect of diagnosis, investigation, or treatment.

The 'information' symbol indicates a passage of text that imparts fact(s) that should be remembered.

Assessment of knowledge is by a link to online self-assessment multiple-choice questions, which are marked correct or incorrect, and by short answer questions at the end of the book to which answers are not given because the reader needs to research the topic in the text.

The 'S' symbol (with a number) indicates a link to the flowcharts which can be found at the end of the book in Appendix I.

Chapter 2: Clinical aspects of anatomy, function, pathology, and classification

This chapter deals with the need for a basic understanding of the normal anatomy, physiology, and pathology of the temporomandibular joint and mandibular muscles, which is essential not only for an understanding of the disease processes involved in TMDs but also for an appreciation of treatment objectives.

Chapter 3: Articulatory system examination

This chapter discusses clinical examination and is indispensable! It outlines an easy yet comprehensive examination routine that should be employed for all your patients, not just those with a TMD.

Chapter 4: I've got 'TMJ'

This chapter illustrates a classic history of a common TMD in a patient who thinks that she knows best. This highlights the importance of critical evaluation of the information (baggage) that a patient might bring to the consultation.

Chapter 5: I've got a clicking joint

This represents the most common condition about which you will be asked. Does a click need treatment? This raises your awareness of the need for treatment and the different treatment options for a commonplace complaint.

Chapter 6: I've got a locking joint

Joint locking can be acute or long-standing. Intervention is often necessary, but how and when? The various options are discussed, as is their practical relevance. We explore the range of options from 'doing nothing' to 'surgery'.

Chapter 7: I've got a grating joint

Degenerative joint disease in the temporomandibular joint is very different from disease in the hip. Nature has a part to play, but we can intervene to make life more tolerable for the person with the condition. Learn about the cyclical nature of this condition and its ramifications.

Chapter 8: You've changed my bite

The possibility of introducing iatrogenic changes to a patient's bite is quite real and can have immediate consequences. Avoidance of the problem is the best approach but to do this you must be aware of the potential pitfalls in restorative care.

Chapter 9: I've got pain in my face

Differential diagnosis is often a complex procedure but must not be avoided. You must avoid tunnel vision and keep an open mind about a patient's complaint no matter how badly explained or difficult to follow. Facial pain is a minefield of potential diagnoses and must be approached logically.

Chapter 10: I've got a dislocated jaw

Although true dislocation is rare, immediate action gives your patient (and you) the best chance of resolving the problem. Learn how to differentiate dislocation from other conditions and how to manage the acute case.

Chapter 11: My teeth are worn

Management of tooth surface loss is a complex treatment, but some straightforward rules will help in diagnosis of the cause, monitoring of the situation, and its management.

Chapter 12: I've got a headache

Headache is a very complex condition even to diagnose. The relationship of headache to TMD is explored, as is the role of the dentist in treating patients whose primary complaint is headache.

Chapter 13: I've got whiplash

Nowadays litigation, especially in relation to road traffic accidents, is commonplace. TMD can be caused by a 'whiplash-type' injury. Make sure that your examination of such a patient is comprehensive and that you are able to produce the necessary records on demand. Be aware that a TMD can become apparent immediately after an accident as well as becoming evident some time later.

Chapter 14: What's of use to me in practice?

You must be aware of what is available and useful in general practice. There is little point in a costly treatment plan being developed if the patient cannot afford it. Similarly provision of a splint that you know your patient will not wear is pointless. This gives guidelines towards accessing the best treatment for your patient and when to employ it.

Chapter 15: You and the lawyer

Litigation is never too far away! Although you should not practise 'litigation dentistry' because this is not in your patient's best interests, you should be aware of the common pitfalls. Above all else maintain good records and good communication, and do not over-reach your abilities.

Chapter 16: The referral letter

A good referral letter is of great help to the specialist. A poor referral letter is a waste of everyone's time and can, on occasion, be embarrassing for all.

Chapter 17: How to make a splint

This is a 'how-to-do' chapter. It is important for you to know what the technician does from impression taking to delivering the splint back to you ready for insertion and fitting. The patient will often ask about this and appreciate an explanation.

Chapter 18: Bruxism: Current knowledge of aetiology and management

This chapter deals with the most updated information about the postulated theories of aetiology and management of bruxism. New definitions and outcomes of recent international consensus are always discussed.

Chapter 19: Splint therapy for the management of TMD patients: An evidence-based approach

The effectiveness of splint therapy for the management of TMD and Bruxism have been discussed in this chapter. The results of the most updated randomized controlled trials and systematic review have been discussed.

Chapter 20: Patient information

This chapter contains general patient information, in template form, that you might like to use for imparting patient advice when appropriate.

Appendix I: Flowcharts

This chapter contains 13 flowcharts which summarise some essential concepts in the management of a TMD. A reference for each relevant chart has been indicated in the text.

Appendix II: Glossary of terms

This is more of a dictionary of terms than merely a glossary of terms used in this book. This provides the reader with a 'TMD and occlusion' dictionary.

This chapter identifies the relevant terms from the glossary of prosthodontic terms published regularly in the *Journal of Prosthetic Dentistry*. Additional terms are added from the book *A Clinical Guide to Temporomandibular Disorders*, BDJ Publications, 1997.

Appendix III: Short answer questions

This chapter includes short answer questions for the reader to practise. The knowledge gained from reading this book will enable the reader to answer these questions effectively.

There is a unique link to an online interactive multiple-choice question (MCQ) site at www.wiley.com/go/al-ani/temporomandibular-disorders-2e. This quiz aims to test your knowledge of TMD and to make reading this book more enjoyable, stimulating, and productive.

Chapter 2

Clinical Aspects of Anatomy, Function, Pathology, and Classification

The joint anatomy, histology, structure, capsule, synovial membrane, and fluid, ligaments

The articulatory system comprises the temporomandibular joints (TMJs) and, intra-articular discs, mandibular/jaw muscles and occlusion.

In the simplest terms, the temporomandibular joint is the articulation between the upper and lower jaws. The teeth form the contacts between the upper and lower jaws, and the muscles are the motors that move the mandible. This system is unique in that the TMJs are paired; any stimulus that affects one joint or any other single part of the articulatory system can have a 'knock-on effect' in the rest of the system.

It is important to have an understanding of anatomy not only to be able to differentiate between what is physiological and what is pathological but also to understand the objectives of some treatment options.

The TMJ (Figure 2.1) is a synovial diarthrodial joint, which means that the joint is lubricated by synovial fluid, and the joint space is divided into two separate compartments by means of an intra-articular disc. The movements that take place in the compartments are predominantly a sliding movement in the upper joint space between the upper surface of the disc and the inferior surface of the glenoid fossa, and a rotational movement in the lower joint space between the head of the condyle and the undersurface of the intra-articular disc. Unlike the articular surfaces of other synovial joints, where the surfaces are typically lined by hyaline cartilage, the articular surface of the TMJ is covered by a layer of fibrocartilagenous tissue. It was thought that this arrangement reflected a non-load bearing functional role for the TMJ; however, a more likely explanation is that, because the covering layer of the condyle is derived

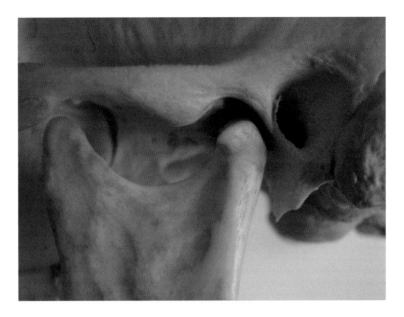

Figure 2.1 The temporomandibular joint (M. Ziad Al-Ani, Robin J.M. Gray.)

from intramembranous ossification, rather than endochondrol ossification, it therefore lacks the endochondrol template from which hyaline articular cartilage is derived.

Histology

There are four distinct layers or zones described in the articular surface of the condyle and mandibular fossa. These layers are the articular zone, proliferative zone, cartilagenous zone, and calcified zone (Figure 2.2):

1. The articular zone is dense fibrous connective tissue and forms the outer functional surface of the condyle head. As a result of this fibrous connective tissue layer, it is suggested that it is less susceptible to the effect of ageing and breakdown over time. In addition, despite a poor blood supply, it has a better ability to repair, good adaptation to sliding movement, and the ability to act as a shock absorber when compared with hyaline cartilage.
2. The proliferative zone is mainly cellular and is the area in which undifferentiated germinative mesenchyme cells are found. This layer is responsible for the proliferation of the articular cartilage and the proliferative zone is capable of regenerative activity and differentiation throughout life.
3. The cartilagenous zone contains collagen fibres arranged in a criss-cross pattern of bundles. This offers considerable resistance against compressive and lateral forces but becomes thinner with age.

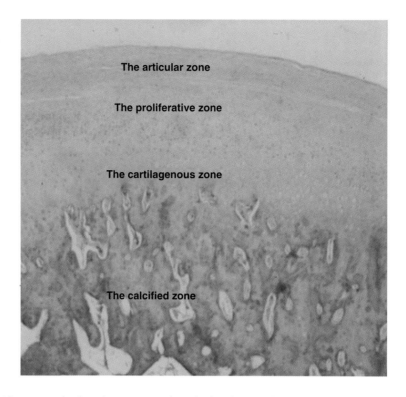

The articular zone

The proliferative zone

The cartilagenous zone

The calcified zone

Figure 2.2 The four distinct zones described in the articular surface of the condyle and mandibular fossa (M. Ziad Al-Ani, Robin J.M. Gray.)

4. The calcified zone is the deepest zone and is made up of chondrocytes, chondroblasts, and osteoblasts. This is an active site for remodelling activity as bone growth proceeds.

The joint capsule

The joint capsule (Figure 2.3) envelops the articular disc and is attached superiorly to the rim of the glenoid fossa and articular eminence and inferiorly to the neck of the condyle. Posteriorly it is attached to the bilaminar zone and anteriorly becomes continuous with the pterygoid muscle attachment. Although it is thin both anteriorly and posteriorly, it is strengthened laterally by the lateral temporomandibular ligament which is not a discrete ligament but a thickened part of the capsule.

Synovial membrane

The glistening inner surface of the capsule comprises the synovial membrane. At birth, this membrane covers all internal joint surfaces but is lost from articular surfaces as function commences. The flexibility of the inner

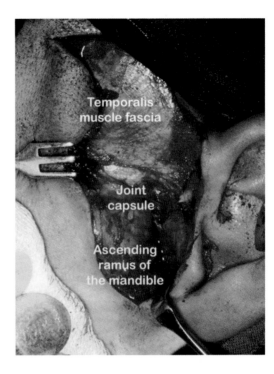

Figure 2.3 The joint capsule (M. Ziad Al-Ani, Robin J.M. Gray.)

surface of the capsule is increased by finger-like projections (villi) of the synovial membrane which disperse the synovial fluid.

The function of the synovial membrane is considered to be

- regulatory because it controls electrolyte balance and nutrients
- secretory via the interstitial cells
- phagocytic.

Synovial fluid is a clear, pale-yellow, viscous solution secreted by the synovial tissues and consists mainly of an ultrafiltrate of plasma enriched with a proteoglycan-containing hyaluronic acid synthesised by synovial cells. The high viscosity of this fluid is a result of the presence of sodium hyaluronate which provides lubrication. The synovial fluid also allows removal of degradation products from the joint space, lubrication of the joint surfaces, and nutrition of the vascular parts of the joint.

Ligaments

The temporomandibular ligament

The temporomandibular ligament is a strong band of fibrous tissue originating as a thickening of the lateral aspect of the joint capsule. It starts at

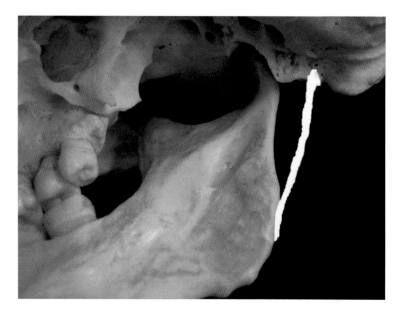

Figure 2.4 The position of stylomandibular ligament. (M. Ziad Al-Ani, Robin J.M. Gray.)

the root of the zygoma and passes obliquely towards the posterior margin of the neck of the condyle, blending into the joint capsule. In the rest position, this ligament is relaxed, but it is thought that, during retrusive and protrusive movements of the condyle, it limits movement in an anteroposterior direction.

The stylomandibular ligament

This is considered as an accessory ligament. It is a specialised band of cervical fibrous tissue extending from the styloid process to the medial border of the mandible at its angle (Figure 2.4). The function of this ligament is not clear but it is thought to limit anteroposterior movements of the mandible.

The sphenomandibular ligament

This ligament is also considered to be accessory. It comprises a flat band of fibrous tissue originating from the spine of the sphenoid bone and passes down to its insertion at the inferior margin of the mandibular foramen (lingula) (Figure 2.5). Again, its function is not certain, but it is thought to limit lateral condylar movements.

The intra-articular disc (meniscus)

About 55 years ago, Rees described the intra-articular disc as being like a 'school-boy's cap'. It is an oval-shaped tense sheet of fibrous

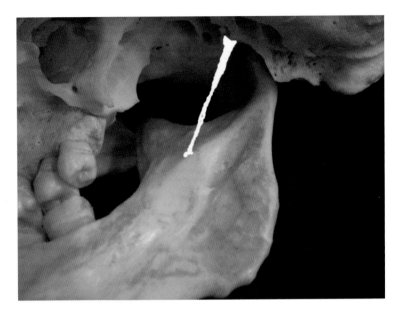

Figure 2.5 The position of sphenomandibular ligament. (M. Ziad Al-Ani, Robin J.M. Gray.)

tissue with a concave inferior surface sitting on the head of the condyle (Figure 2.6). On its posterior aspect, it has a convex upper surface; it becomes saddle-shaped on its anterior aspect. It overlays the condylar head and blends medially and laterally with the capsule. It is also attached to the medial and lateral poles of the condyle and anteriorly to the superior pterygoid muscle. This structural arrangement, as it is interposed between the head of the condyle and the glenoid fossa, divides the joint into the upper and lower joint spaces (Figure 2.7).

There are four zones of the disc:

1. The anterior band which is of moderate thickness but narrow in an anteroposterior direction.
2. The intermediate band, which is the thinnest zone of the disc.
3. The posterior band, which is both the thickest and the widest transverse zone of the disc.
4. The bilaminar zone, which consists of two parts: the superior band, which is attached to the posterior wall of the glenoid fossa and squamotympanic fissure and is elastic, and the inferior band, which is attached to the neck of the condyle and is fibrous.

The disc is attached anteriorly to the margin of the articular eminence superiorly and to the articular margin of the condyle inferiorly. Posteriorly, the disc is attached to the glenoid fossa and squamotympanic fissure

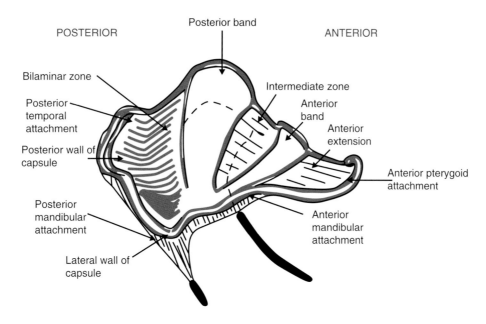

Figure 2.6 Diagram of disc morphology. (Rees LA. The structure and function of the mandibular joint. J Br Dent Assoc 1954; XCVI:126–33.)

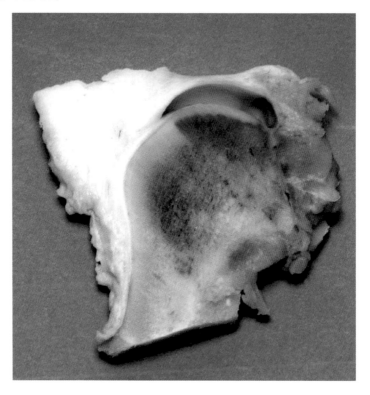

Figure 2.7 Sagittal section of porcine temporomandibular joint. As in human beings, the articular surface of the mandibular condyle is convex and joins the lower articular surface of the meniscus, which is concave, to form a condylomeniscal joint. (M. Ziad Al-Ani, Robin J.M. Gray.)

(elastic attachment) and to the distal aspect of the neck of the condyle (fibrous attachment). This is termed the 'posterior bilaminar zone'. Medially and laterally the meniscus blends with the capsule. The disc is also attached to adjacent muscles, namely the lateral pterygoid (anteriorly) and masseter and temporalis muscles (laterally). The fibres of the lateral pterygoid muscle merge with the disc anteriorly to form its true insertion. The connections with the masseter and temporalis muscles are less strong, consisting of fibrous bands of thickened tissue at right angles to the direction of the muscle fibres.

This varying thickness of the bands in the disc is significant when considering the functional anatomy of the joint. The meniscus is flexible and able to alter shape to concave or convex during forward movement of the condyle, because of the thinner intermediate zone between the two thicker anterior and posterior zones.

In the "at rest" mandibular position, the condyle is separated from the temporal bone by the thick posterior band. As the head of the condyle moves forward towards the articular eminence, it is separated from the temporal bone by the thinner intermediate zone and, as anterior movement progresses, the head of the condyle continues to move forwards until it is resting on the thicker but narrow anterior band.

During mouth opening, the disc moves forwards but not to the same extent or with the same speed as the head of the condyle. The forward movement of the meniscus is permitted by the loose fibroelastic tissue of the bilaminar zone, which is stretchable to 7–10 mm. In addition, the structures of the bilaminar zone are ideally suited to filling the void of the vacated glenoid fossa when the condyle is in a protrusive position.

The non-elastic lower band attached to the posterior neck of the condyle contributes to the return of the meniscus during retrusion of the mandible. This is helped by the elastic recoil of the upper attachment.

The disc acts as a 'shock absorber' during masticatory function. The central part of the disc is mainly avascular and depends on nutrition from diffusion from the synovial fluid. A rich vascular plexus is, however, present in the posterior part of the bilaminar zone which is mainly supplied from the deep auricular artery, a branch of the internal maxillary artery. Although the central part of the meniscus is poorly innervated, the bilaminar zone has a dense innervation from a branch of the auricular temporal nerve, the masseteric nerve and the posterior deep temporal nerve.

It has been suggested that the articular disc has many functions which may include shock absorption, increasing congruity between the articular surfaces, allowing combinations of different movements at the joint, ball-bearing action, force distribution by increasing the contact area between articular surfaces, providing stability during mandibular movements and playing a role in assisting joint lubrication by forming thin synovial fluid films.

The bones of the temporomandibular joint

The mandibular condyle

The adult mandibular condyle is roughly elliptical in shape with the largest diameter being mediolateral (Figure 2.8). There is considerable individual variation in both condylar size and angulation to the various planes, and there are often differences between the right and left sides in an individual. The mediolateral dimension varies between 13 and 25 mm and the anteroposterior dimension varies between 6 and 16 mm. The mediolateral angulation to the transverse plane is between 15° and 33° and from 0° to 48° in the horizontal plane. These dimensions vary not only between individuals but between the right and left sides in an individual.

The temporal bone

The articular surface of the temporal bone consists, posteriorly, of the concavity of the glenoid fossa and, anteriorly, of the convexity of the articular eminence; it extends from the anterior margin of the squamo-tympanic fissure to the margin of the articular eminence. The roof of this fossa is very thin, indicating that this part is not a load-bearing area. Anteriorly, however, the articular eminence is thicker and this area, together

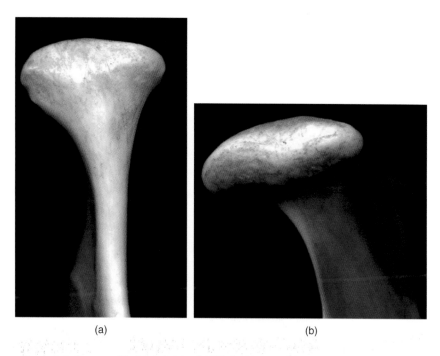

(a)   (b)

Figure 2.8 The mandibular condyle. (M. Ziad Al-Ani, Robin J.M. Gray.)

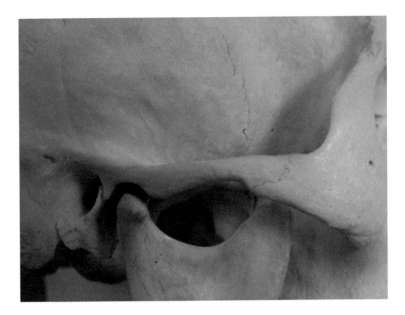

Figure 2.9 The articular part of the temporal bone. (M. Ziad Al-Ani, Robin J.M. Gray.)

with the disc, may be the area that bears most of the load during function (Figure 2.9).

Innervation of the TMJ

This arises from the mandibular division of the trigeminal nerve. The auriculotemporal nerve innervates most of the TMJ mainly anterolaterally and small branches of the masseteric and deep temporal nerves supply the posterior aspect.

Vascular supply to the TMJ

Vascular supply to the TMJ is from the external carotid artery via the internal maxillary artery and the superficial temporal artery.

Mandibular (jaw/masticatory) muscles

The jaw muscles form another component of the articulatory system.

The muscles commonly symptomatic in temporomandibular disorders that are accessible for clinical examination are the masseter, temporalis, lateral pterygoid, and digastric muscles. Other muscles involved but not comprising part of the routine clinical examination are the medial pterygoid, mylohyoid, suprahyoid, infrahyoid, and cervical muscles.

Masseter muscle

This muscle originates from the anterior two-thirds of the zygomatic arch and extends obliquely downwards to its insertion over the lateral surface of the angle of the mandible (Figure 2.10).

Function

There are two portions to this muscle: the superficial and the deep. The superficial masseter is one of the primary elevator muscles of the mandible during jaw closure, but, as some of its fibres are angled anteriorly, it also assists in protrusion of the mandible. The deep portion is one of the main elevators of the mandible but, as some of its fibres run posteriorly, it is active in retrusion of the mandible.

Parafunction

This muscle is active during clenching of the teeth and is frequently found to be tender at its origin and less frequently at its insertion.

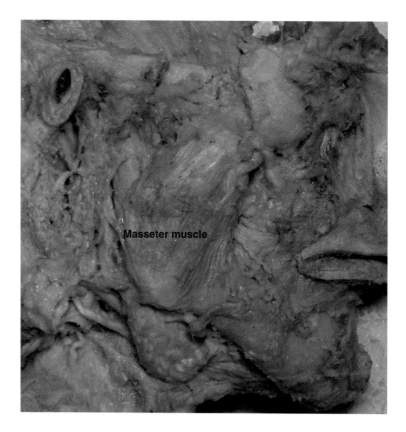

Figure 2.10 The masseter muscle. (Figure courtesy of Dr Paul Rea and Caroline Morris, University of Glasgow.)

Examination

The muscle is examined bimanually with one finger inside and one finger outside the mouth to palpate the origin and insertion of this muscle. It is usually tender where it inserts into bone (Chapter 3).

The temporalis muscle

This is a large, broad, fan-shaped muscle that has its origin in the temporal fossa between the superior and inferior temporal lines, which run across the parietal bone, temporal bone, and greater wing of the sphenoid, extending forwards to the temporal surface of the frontal bone. The fibres of this muscle run in various directions and converge into a tendinous insertion which runs under the zygomatic arch and inserts into the coronoid process and anterior border of the ascending ramus of the mandible (Figure 2.11).

Function

The anterior fibres of this muscle, which form its major bulk, are mainly vertical and elevators of the mandible. Progressing posteriorly along the middle and posterior parts of the muscle, the fibres become increasingly oblique and the posterior fibres are almost horizontal. The anterior fibres are elevators of the mandible. The posterior fibres retrude the mandible.

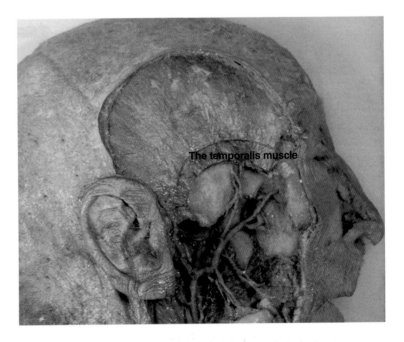

Figure 2.11 The temporalis muscle. (Figure courtesy of Dr Paul Rea and Caroline Morris, University of Glasgow.)

Parafunction

In parafunction, this muscle becomes symptomatic and painful, usually in the anterior part of the temple, in patients who perform the parafunctional activity of bruxism or tooth grinding.

Examination

This muscle is accessible to digital palpation only over its origin. It is usually the anterior vertical fibres that are tender to digital palpation, although the posterior horizontal fibres can on occasion also be found to be tender. The insertion of this muscle is not accessible for digital palpation (Chapter 3).

The lateral pterygoid muscle

Controversy still surrounds this muscle as to whether it has one single or two separate heads and one single or two different actions. It is, however, generally regarded that the lateral pterygoid muscle has two separate parts, these being the inferior belly and the superior belly usually referred to as the superior and inferior pterygoids. The inferior pterygoid originates in the lateral surface of the lateral pterygoid plate and inserts into a fossa in the anterior part of the head of the condyle. The superior pterygoid originates from the infratemporal surface of the greater wing of the sphenoid bone and inserts into the anterior part of the capsule and intra-articular disc. It also has a small attachment into the fossa in the anterior part of the head of the condyle (Figure 2.12).

Function

The function of this muscle is thought to be twofold: first, it assists in opening the mouth and in depression of the mandible; second it assists in protrusion of the mandible and lateral movements. In addition, this muscle is thought to be important in stabilisation of the condyle/intra-articular disc/fossa assembly.

There is controversy about the precise action of the pterygoid muscle. However, it is clear that this is an important muscle in protrusion of the mandible, which occurs when both right and left muscles act synchronously. When the pterygoid muscle on one side contracts, the effect is to pull the mandible laterally towards that side.

Parafunction

In parafunction, there appears to be increased activity in both superior and inferior pterygoids which appears to cause pain referred to the preauricular region when the muscle is examined against resistance. In addition,

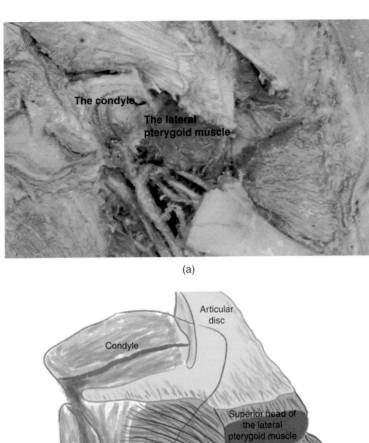

(a)

(b)

Figure 2.12 The lateral pterygoid muscle (a) (Courtesy of Dr Paul Rea and Caroline Morris, University of Glasgow.) (b) Schematic representation illustrating the insertion of the superior and inferior heads of the lateral pterygoid muscle (capsule cut away).

it is thought possible that sustained tonic contraction of the superior pterygoid muscle can be a factor in anteromedial displacement of the intra-articular disc.

Examination

This muscle is not accessible to digital palpation and should be examined against resistance. The patient should be asked to open the mouth to a certain point; the operator's hand is then placed under the chin and resistance is applied by the examiner. If there is lateral pterygoid tenderness discomfort will be felt in the preauricular region. In addition, this muscle can be examined by resisting lateral movements. The patient should slide the jaw across to one side and the operator applies resistance to this lateral movement. If there is lateral pterygoid tenderness, pain in the contralateral side to the pressure will be elicited (Chapter 3).

Medial pterygoid muscle

This muscle arises from the medial surface of the lateral pterygoid plate and the lateral aspect of the medial pterygoid plate and inserts into the angle of the mandible on the medial surface opposite the insertion of the masseter (Figure 2.13).

Function

The action of this muscle is elevation of the mandible, but it also assists in protrusion and lateral excursions of the mandible.

Parafunction

This is not a muscle that can be reliably examined clinically so the effect of parafunction on the muscle is just conjecture.

Examination

The medial pterygoid muscle is not accessible for manual or digital palpation.

Cervical muscles

These are many muscles including the digastric, mylohyoid, geniohyoid, and stylohyoid muscles (Figure 2.14).

The two muscles in this group that mainly merit consideration are the digastric and mylohyoid muscles. The digastric muscle has two separate parts: an anterior and posterior belly; the two bellies have quite different

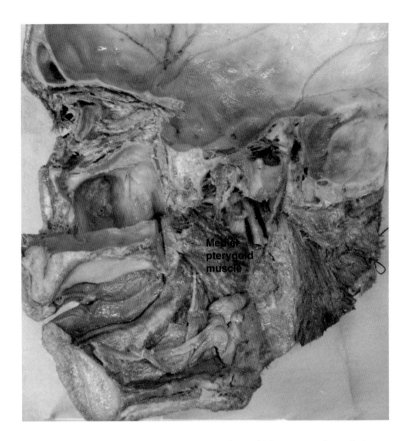

Figure 2.13 Medial pterygoid showing ramus of mandible sectioned: medial pterygoid muscle. (Figure courtesy of Dr Paul Rea and Caroline Morris, University of Glasgow.)

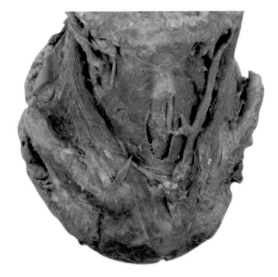

Figure 2.14 Cervical muscles. (Figure courtesy of Dr Paul Rea and Caroline Morris, University of Glasgow.)

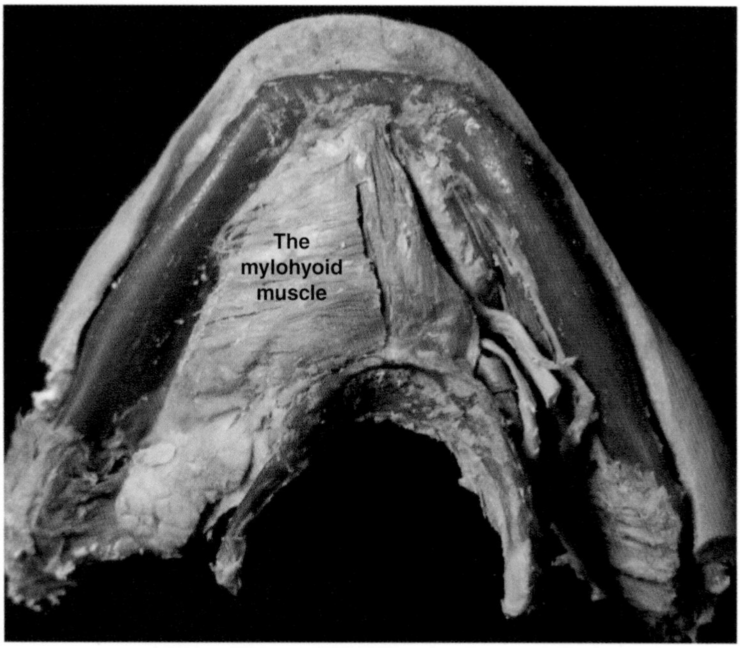

Figure 2.15 The mylohyoid muscle. (Figure courtesy of Dr Paul Rea and Caroline Morris, University of Glasgow.)

actions. They are connected by an intermediate tendon that runs through a fibrous sling on the hyoid bone.

The mylohyoid muscle is a thin sheet of muscle arising on the inner aspect of the mandible from the whole length of the mylohyoid line. The two halves of this muscle meet in a median raphe, which inserts into the body of the hyoid bone. This muscle forms the floor of the mouth, separates the submandibular and sublingual regions, and is unattached posteriorly (Figure 2.15).

Function

The suprahyoid muscles raise the hyoid bone and the larynx. They can also depress the mandible together with the tongue and the floor of the mouth, but only when the infrahyoid muscles stabilise the hyoid bone. The posterior belly of the digastric is, in addition one of the retruding muscles of the mandible.

This group of muscles also acts to depress the hyoid bone and larynx during swallowing. The infrahyoid and suprahyoid muscles always contract bilaterally (Figure 2.16).

Parafunction

There is little evidence to directly link the suprahyoid muscles to parafunctional symptoms apart from the digastric muscle. This muscle is found to

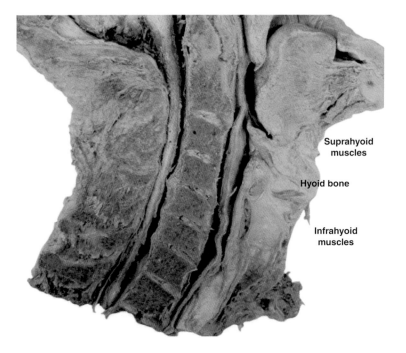

Figure 2.16 The infrahyoid and suprahyoid muscles. (Courtesy of Dr Paul Rea and Caroline Morris, University of Glasgow.)

be tender either behind the ascending ramus of the mandible or in the submandibular region in patients who have a parafunctional bruxist habit, which they perform on their anterior teeth.

Examination

Tenderness in the posterior and/or anterior belly of the digastric can be recorded by digital palpation. In this instance, discomfort can be elicited by palpating behind the ascending ramus of the mandible or in the submandibular area below the body of the mandible. Tenderness in this muscle arises in patients who demonstrate bruxism on their anterior teeth with the mandible in protrusion.

The other suprahyoid, infrahyoid, and cervical muscles are difficult to examine apart from sternocleidomastoid, which can be examined by asking the patient to place the chin towards the shoulder and palpating the origin and insertion of the muscle on the opposite side.

Sternocleidomastoid muscle

The sternocleidomastoid muscle has two heads, one originating in the sternum and one in the clavicle; insertion of this muscle is into the mastoid process. When the sternocleidomastoid muscles act together they flex the

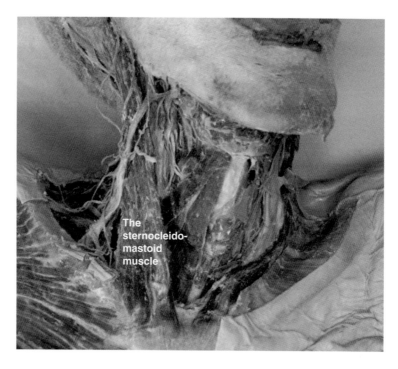

Figure 2.17 The sternocleidomastoid muscle. (Courtesy of Dr Paul Rea and Caroline Morris, University of Glasgow.)

neck. When one acts on its own it flexes the neck laterally and rotates the head.

These are important muscles to consider if your patient has, for instance, had a whiplash cervical extension/flexion injury and complains of generalised facial and cervical spine pain (Figure 2.17).

Classification and Pathology

When considering temporomandibular disorders by frequency of presentation, pathological changes within the joint complex are relatively uncommon. Let us consider the disorders divided by frequency of presentation into rare, uncommon and common conditions. We confine this script to the clinical relevance of pathological changes. Definitive text on pathology can be found elsewhere.

Rare conditions

Rare conditions that affect the TMJ are very rare indeed. There are two conditions that you might encounter: condylar hyperplasia and neoplasms (benign and malignant).

Condylar hyperplasia

The undifferentiated germinative mesenchyme cell layer persists in the mandibular condyle throughout life. This is one of the primary growth centres of the jaw in adolescence. There are three presentations of condylar hyperplasia. The first is when, during the pubertal growth spurt, one growth centre is more active than the other, and this results in a facial and occlusal irregularity where the asymmetry is vertical; the second is towards the end of puberty when one growth centre 'switches off' when the other does not. The clinical presentation of this is a combined vertical and horizontal facial asymmetry. The third is when the growth centre on one side becomes active, but the other side is inactive; this produces a horizontal discrepancy and facial asymmetry.

Neoplasms

Tumours are rare, but ostoesarcoma and chondrosarcoma do present. Metastatic carcinoma is the most frequently occurring malignancy; however, the jaws are an uncommon site for metastasis, especially the mandibular condyle. When considering benign tumours, osteochondroma is the most common, but this is still very rare (Figure 2.18).

Features that may suggest the possibility of a tumour in the TMJ include pain, swelling, paraesthesia, trismus, and occlusal changes. There may rarely be auditory changes secondary to eighth nerve involvement.

Use of radiographs and other imaging studies is of diagnostic importance and surgery is the treatment. The pathology depends on the diagnosis of the tumour.

Uncommon conditions

Uncommon conditions affecting the TMJ include rheumatoid arthritis and psoriatic arthritis. Pathologically there is a thickened synovial membrane and joint effusion. There is cartilage destruction and cortical erosion and, in advanced stages of both diseases, severe bone destruction or proliferation may occur (Figure 2.19); on very rare occasions fibrous or bony ankylosis can be the end-point. If there is severe osteolysis, destruction of a condylar head can occur and an anterior open bite may result. It is not normal for a patient to present with rheumatoid or psoriatic arthritis in the TMJ as the first symptom. Usually diagnosis of the systemic disease will have preceded this late involvement.

Common conditions

When considering the common disorders of the TMJ, myofascial pain, (facial arthromyalgia/pain dysfunction syndrome), internal derangements, osteoarthrosis, and the response to trauma, the tissue changes are primarily inflammatory except in osteoarthrosis.

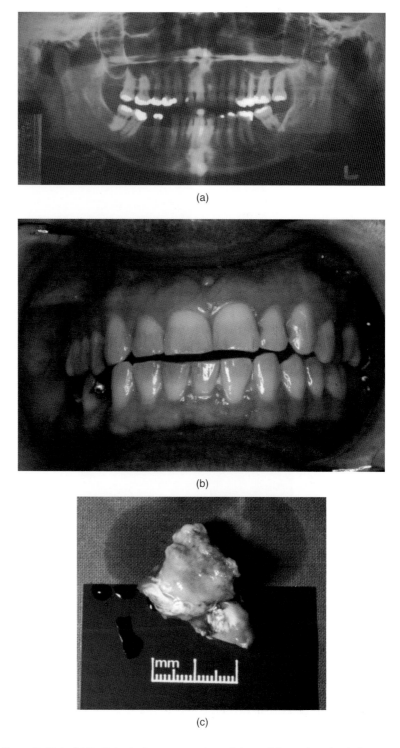

(a)

(b)

(c)

Figure 2.18 (a, b) Radiological (mass anterior to left condyle) and occlusal changes (anterior open bite and midline deviation to the right) in a patient with osteochondroma in the left temporomandibular joint. (c) The tumour surgically removed. (M. Ziad Al-Ani, Robin J.M. Gray.)

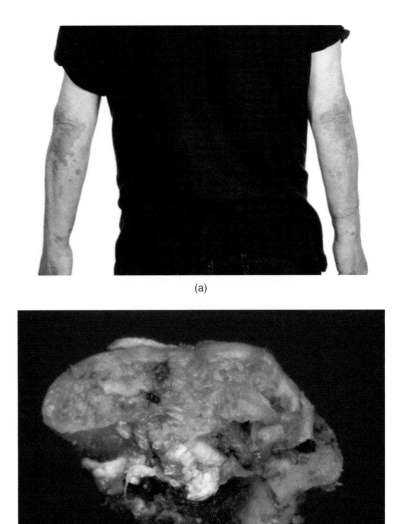

(a)

(b)

Figure 2.19 (a) Psoriasis skin condition; (b) excised condyle of a patient with psoriatic arthritis. (M. Ziad Al-Ani, Robin J.M. Gray.)

Osteoarthrosis is a term that has developed to distinguish between an acute and a chronic condition. Osteoarthrosis describes a non-inflammatory degenerative disease. In osteoarthrosis, the disorder appears to be primarily degenerative, starting with changes within the bone and progressing through the surface tissues of the joint to subsequent involve degeneration of the articulatory surface and formation of erosion and eburnation of the surface of, usually, the mandibular condyle. These changes can also be seen, however, in the articulatory fossa (glenoid fossa). The difference therefore between osteo-'arthritis' and osteo-'arthrosis' is that the former is first recognised in the fluid surrounding the joint which then permeates the hard structures, whereas the latter starts in the hard structures permeating through the surfaces of the joint. From a patient's point of view, the encouraging feature is that, as the germinative mesenchyme cell layer remains throughout life, this can respond, as a result of 'irritation', to produce new tissue. Therefore, it is not uncommon for a patient who presents with osteoarthrosis of the TMJ to enter a phase of acute symptoms followed by a plateau stage followed by improvement of symptoms as remodelling and resurfacing of the condyle progress.

The clinical symptoms of osteoarthrosis include pain localised to the joint and limited movement which is worse with function. The clinical joint sound is crepitation, which is a grating or crunching sound from the joint that indicates a loss of the smooth articular surfaces. Crepitation can emanate from the articulating surfaces or the disc.

Disc displacement

A further pathological change is related to disc displacement (DD) if the intra-articular disc is anteromedially displaced. The highly innervated posterior part of the bilaminar zone, which contains elastic fibers can, with the passage of time, undergo morphological changes that render this part of the disc more fibrous. It has been reported that cartilaginous changes can also occur in this situation, which is associated with long-standing DD when the initial symptoms would have included pain due to compression of this innervated tissue. The pain gradually diminishes as the tissue undergoes the aforementioned morphological changes of conversion from innervated elastic to less innervated fibrous tissue.

Myofascial pain

In the case of myofascial pain, there is no readily demonstrable histopathology.

Diagnoses of TMDs

There is a multitude of classifications based upon the aetiology, clinical signs and symptoms, or anatomy; all have their weaknesses. Those classification systems that define the different kinds of TMD and utilize the history and examination provide the most help to the general dental practitioner as well as to the researcher.

The gold standard classification system for research is currently the TMD research diagnostic criteria (RDC/TMD).

This is a dual axis classification of TMD pain in a research tool which aims to provide a more rational, scientific basis for TMD diagnosis.

Axis 1: a set of opertionalised RDC for use in evaluating and investigating masticatory muscle pain, DD and degenerative diseases of the TMJ.

Axis 2: a set of operational RDC to assess chronic pain, dysfunction, depression, non-specific physical symptoms, and orofacial disability.

The RDC categorise TMD criteria into three groups according to the common factors among conditions.

GROUP I: Muscle disorders

I.a Myofascial pain
  Criteria: Reported pain in masticatory muscles
  Pain on palpation in at least three sites, one of them at least in the same side of the reported pain.
I.b Myofascial pain with limited opening
  Criteria: Myofascial pain
  Pain-free unassisted opening <40 mm and passive stretch ≥5 mm.

GROUP II: DDs

II.a DD with reduction
  Criteria: No pain in the joint
  Reproducible click on excursion with either opening or closing click
  With click on opening and closing (unless excursive click confirmed):
  - Click on opening occurs at ≥5 mm interincisal distance than on closing
  - Clicks eliminated by protrusive opening
II.b DD without reduction with limited opening
  Criteria: History of locking or catching that interfered with eating
  Absence of TMJ clicking
  Unassisted opening (even painful) ≤35 mm and passive stretch ≤4 mm
  Contralateral excursion <7 mm or uncorrected ipsilateral deviation on opening
II.c DD without reduction without limited opening
  Criteria: History of locking or catching that interfered with eating
  The presence of TMJ sounds excluding DDR clicking
  Unassisted opening (even painful) >35 mm and passive stretch >4 mm
  Contralateral excursion ≥7 mm 5. Optional imaging (Arthrography or MRI) to confirm DD

GROUP III: Other common joint disorders

III.a Arthralgia
    Pain and tenderness/no crepitation
       Criteria: Pain on TMJ palpation either laterally or intra auricular
       Self-reported joint pain with or without jaw movement
       Absence of crepitus, and possibility of clicking
III.b Osteoarthritis
    Inflammatory condition
    Pain
    Crepitation and/or changes on radiograph
       Criteria: Pain as for arthralgia
       Crepitus on any movement or radiographic evidence of joint changes
III.c Osteoarthrosis
    Degenerative disorder
    No pain
    Crepitation and/or changes on radiograph
       Criteria: Crepitus on any movement or radiographic evidence of joint changes
       No reported joint pain nor pain on any movement

Further Reading

Avery, J. (2006). *Essential of Oral Histology and Embryology: A Clinical Approach*, 3nde. St Louis, MO: Mosby.

Gage, J.P. (1989). Mechanisms of disc displacement in the temporomandibular joint. *Aust Dent J* 34: 427–436.

Gray, R.J., Davies, S.J., and Quayle, A.A. (1994). A clinical approach to temporomandibular disorders. 1. Classification and functional anatomy. *Br Dent J* 176: 429–435.

Rees, L.A. (1954). The structure and function of the mandibular joint. *J Br Dent Assoc* XCVI: 126–133.

Schiffman, E., Ohrbach, R., Truelove, E. et al. (2014). Diagnostic criteria for temporomandibular disorders (DC/TMD) for clinical and research applications: recommendations of the international RDC/TMD consortium network and orofacial pain special interest group. *J Oral Facial Pain Headache* 28: 6–27.

Chapter 3

Articulatory System Examination

Examination of the articulatory system should be a routine that you perform for all new patients and at regular intervals for existing patients, even those whom you know well. Symptoms of a temporomandibular disorder can come and go, and the patient may present complaining of the recent onset of a symptom such as a click which, by chance, was not present at the time of your previous examination. The three components to examine are the temporomandibular joints (TMJs), the mandibular muscles, and the occlusion.

3.1 Examination of the temporomandibular joints

Range of movement

Examination of the range of movement involves examining the interincisal opening, both pain-free and maximum (Figure 3.1) and lateral excursions of the mandible.

The lower limit of normal range of incisal opening is regarded as being approximately 35 mm for female patients and 42 mm for male patients. The opening is usually measured from incisal tip to incisal tip. It does not matter whether or not the overbite is included in your measurement regimen as long as you are always consistent in either including the overbite or excluding it so that your measurements are comparable and reproducible.

The range of lateral mandibular excursions (lower limit 8 mm on either side) should be measured from upper incisal midline to lower midline, with the patient moving the mandible first to one side then to the other (Figure 3.2).

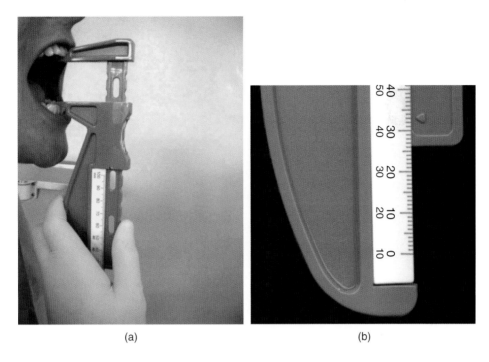

(a)   (b)

Figure 3.1 Measurement of incisal opening. (M. Ziad Al-Ani, Robin J.M. Gray.)

Any starting discrepancy in the incisal midlines when the patient is in centric occlusion should be taken into account.

Pathway of jaw opening

Stand in front of your patient and ask him or her to repeatedly open and close the mouth as far as comfortably possible. Carefully watch the pathway and range of jaw movement. You can learn a lot from looking!

The mandible can open in a straight pathway or with a transient or lasting deviation. The mandibular pathway can be observed by standing in front of the patient and asking the patient to repeatedly open and close the mouth. Limitation or deviation of mandibular movement can be caused by two principal factors: either pain in the mandibular muscles or TMJ, or a physical obstruction to movement. Much can be gained from examining the patient slowly opening and closing the mouth (Figure 3.3).

If the pathway is straight throughout the whole range of mandibular movement, this indicates that both joints are acting synchronously (Figure 3.3a).

If there is a deviation to one side and then back to the midline, or alternatively first to one side then across to the other and back to the midline, with the mandibular incisal midline coinciding with the maxillary incisal midline at maximum opening, this would imply that there has been a

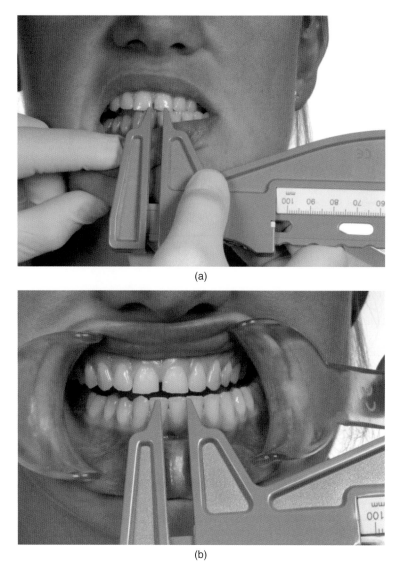

(a)

(b)

Figure 3.2 Measurement of lateral jaw movement. (M. Ziad Al-Ani, Robin J.M. Gray.)

temporary obstruction to smooth mandibular movement, possibly due to disc displacement with reduction (Figure 3.3b).

If the mandible moves obliquely from the start of the opening cycle to the end of the opening cycle, this may imply that there are adhesions within the joint, with one condyle moving less well than the other throughout the range of movement (Figure 3.3c).

If the mandible moves vertically during the first phase of movement and then has an abrupt lateral deviation, this could imply that there is disc displacement without reduction. In this instance, the mouth opens normally until the head of the condyle on the affected side encounters the disc in the unexpected and displaced position. Further translation of

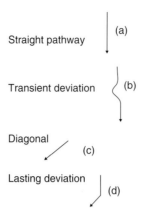

Figure 3.3 Diagrammatic representation of mandibular movements.

the condyle is prevented, thereby resulting in marked lateral deviation (Figure 3.3d).

Let us now consider the features of lateral movements. If there is disc displacement without reduction on one side and not the other, let us assume that this is the right side; the patient will be able to move the mandible to the right very much more freely than to the left because, on right lateral excursion, the right condyle pivots in the fossa and lateral jaw movement is attainable. If, however, as is usually the case, the intra-articular disc is displaced anteromedially, lateral movements of the mandible to the left side will be reduced because the condylar movement will be blocked by the disc, thereby severely limiting mandibular excursion in this direction.

Maxillary and mandibular midlines

If a patient has a straight pathway or transient mandibular deviation during opening, then at maximum opening the upper and lower midlines will coincide (Figure 3.4). In the case of a patient with disc displacement without reduction, the maxillary and mandibular incisal midlines will remain coincident until the point at which the head of the condyle encounters the displaced disc and a lateral shift will then occur. There will then be an obvious discrepancy between the upper and lower centre lines at maximum opening (Figure 3.5).

When there are adhesions in the joint, either between the disc and fossa or the disc and the head of the condyle, then from the start of opening, the maxillary and mandibular incisal centrelines will not coincide.

TMJ tenderness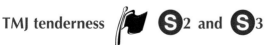

TMJ tenderness can be elicited by different examination techniques: lateral palpation in the immediate preauricular area, intra-auricular

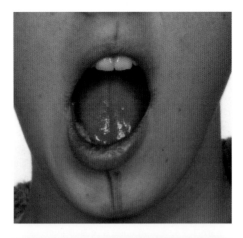

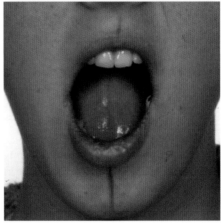

Figure 3.4 (a, b) Transient mandibular deviation during opening. (M. Ziad Al-Ani, Robin J.M. Gray.)

palpation via the external auditory meatus or manipulation of the mandible to a retruded position.

Lateral palpation

The lateral aspect of the joint is palpated by pressing gently over the immediate preauricular area, both at rest and during motion (Figure 3.6).

Tenderness is thought to indicate the presence of inflammation in the capsule. Anatomically, this area is not as well innervated as the posterior part of the joint, and more useful information can be obtained by intra-auricular palpation.

Intra-auricular palpation

TMJ pain and tenderness are mainly related to the area of the posterior bilaminar zone of the disc and the posterior aspect of the capsule.

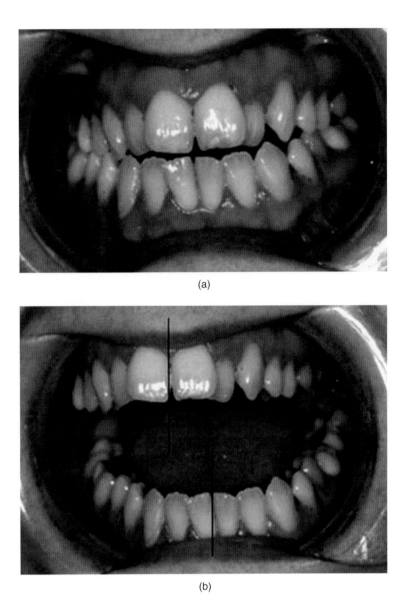

(a)

(b)

Figure 3.5 Lasting deviation to the left. (a) Mouth closed; centre lines coincident. (b) Mouth open; mandibular deviation to the left. (M. Ziad Al-Ani, Robin J.M. Gray.)

Examination of this area can be achieved more readily and reliably by intra-auricular palpation. This involves placing the little finger in the external auditory meatus on one side at a time and applying gentle forward pressure, while asking the patient to open and close the mouth (Figure 3.7).

Be aware that, if there is acute disc displacement, this method of examination can be very uncomfortable for the patient.

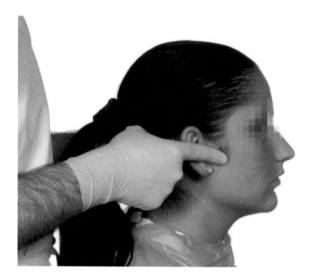

Figure 3.6 Lateral palpation of the temporomandibular joint. (M. Ziad Al-Ani, Robin J.M. Gray.)

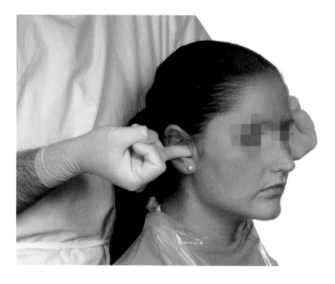

Figure 3.7 Intra-auricular palpation of the temporomandibular joint. (M. Ziad Al-Ani, Robin J.M. Gray.)

Examination by manipulation of the mandible

With the patient relaxed, the mandible is gently manipulated posteriorly by gentle pressure applied to the symphysis region. This is a method of eliciting tenderness in the posterior bilaminar zone by compressing this area of tissue between the distal part of the condyle and the fossa if there is disc displacement. Again, this can be very uncomfortable so only gentle manipulation should be used.

Mandibular (masticatory) muscle tenderness 2

Masseter muscle

This muscle can be palpated bimanually by placing one finger intraorally and another externally on the cheek. The origin of the masseter muscle along the anterior two-thirds of the zygomatic arch is the area frequently found to be tender (Figure 3.8a). There is often a palpable difference between one masseter and the other in that, on the affected side, the muscle tends to be 'bunched up' and quite easy to palpate, whereas on the

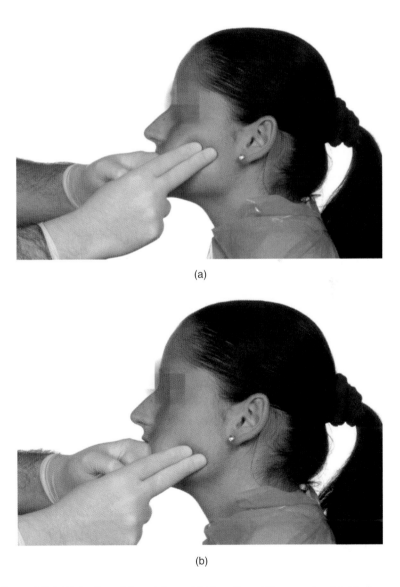

(a)

(b)

Figure 3.8 (a) Palpation of the origin and (b) insertion of the masseter. (M. Ziad Al-Ani, Robin J.M. Gray.)

unaffected side the muscle has a soft rubbery consistency and the margin is less easy to define. The insertion of the masseter on the outer aspect of the angle of the mandible should be palpated (Figure 3.8b), but this is less frequently found to be tender.

Temporalis muscle

This muscle can be examined by palpating its origin extraorally. Ask the patient to clench the teeth together and the outline of the muscle origin can be identified, especially the anterior fibres. Digital palpation can be preformed between the superior and inferior temporal lines extending posteriorly (Figure 3.9).

The anterior, more vertical fibres comprise the main elevator muscle of the jaw and are most commonly tender on palpation. The posterior fibres are almost horizontal in orientation and less frequently tender because their main function is to retrude the mandible.

It is suggested that the insertion of the temporalis muscle into the anterior margin of the coronoid process can be palpated intraorally by placing the little finger on the anterior border of the ramus and running it upwards, but this is not a reliable test because this is an uncomfortable and inaccessible area to try to access even in those who do not have muscle tenderness.

Lateral pterygoid muscle

This muscle is inaccessible to manual palpation so palpation for tenderness lacks validity and reliability and is difficult if not impossible to perform.

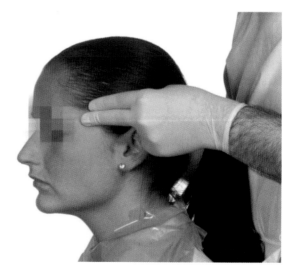

Figure 3.9 Palpation of the anterior vertical fibres of the temporalis. (M. Ziad Al-Ani, Robin J.M. Gray.)

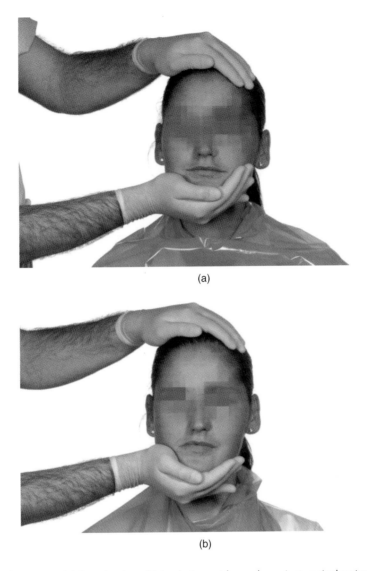

(a)

(b)

Figure 3.10 (a) Examination of lateral pterygoid muscle against vertical resisted movement; (b) Examination of lateral pterygoid muscle against lateral resistance. (M. Ziad Al-Ani, Robin J.M. Gray.)

A more reliable technique is to examine the response to resistance. The patient is asked to open the mouth. The examiner's hand is placed under the patient's chin and pressure is applied to try to close the mouth while the patient tries to resist (Figure 3.10a). This results in a more reliable test because the muscle is fixed. If there is tenderness in the lateral pterygoid muscle, this test will produce pain in the preauricular region. The same can be done by resisting lateral mandibular movement (Figure 3.10b).

If the patient were, for instance to move the mandible to the right and this movement were resisted, left preauricular pain would arise if there was lateral pterygoid tenderness on the left.

Joint sounds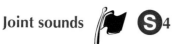

Clicking

Clicking from the TMJ is often felt by the patient but can be inaudible to the examiner. A click can occasionally be felt by palpating the TMJ in the preauricular region but is more often detected on intra-auricular palpation.

If joint sounds are to be listened for, a reliable method is use of a stereo-stethoscope. This consists of a standard earpiece with two outlets, rather than one, and two tubes, each of which is connected to a separate diaphragm (Figure 3.11).

The apparatus provides a method of detecting TMJ sounds and determining whether they emanate from the right or left side or are bilateral. It should be remembered that it is sometimes extremely difficult to determine which side a click is coming from by listening with a stethoscope because of the 'echo' and reverberation across the bones of the skull from the contralateral side. In addition, auscultation permits the clinician to detect the frequently softer closing click that is sometimes difficult to detect on joint palpation alone.

For the diagnosis of disc displacement with reduction and to assist in determining a suitable treatment plan, it is important to determine whether the click can be eliminated by protrusion of the mandible. At the chair side, the patient is asked to protrude the mandible and then perform a series of opening and closing mouth movements, usually with the upper and lower incisors in an 'edge-to-edge' relationship. The click will be present during the first movement but, if the click is eliminated in subsequent movements in this protrusive mandibular position, the diagnosis of disc displacement with reduction is highly probable and it is likely that provision of a suitable splint design will reduce or eliminate the symptoms.

Crepitus

Crepitus is a crunching or grating sound that indicates degenerative joint disease. It can be heard with a stethoscope or, if severe, without when it may be readily audible to others. It can be present throughout the movement cycle or at any point in the cycle.

Signs of bruxism

 Tooth surface loss or tooth wear cannot be taken as a sign that the patient is an **active** bruxist. Even if bruxism is the cause of tooth surface loss, the patient may no longer be performing this parafunctional activity (Figure 3.12a).

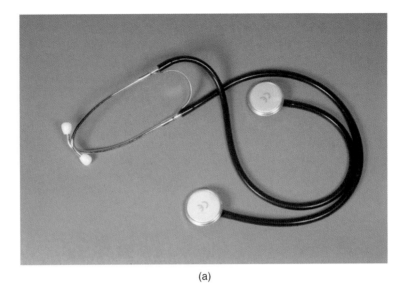

(a)

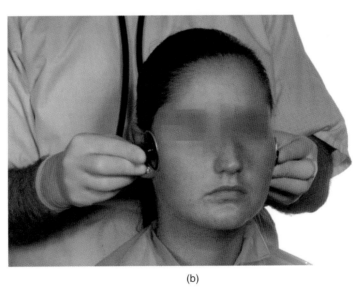

(b)

Figure 3.11 (a) A stereo-stethoscope used for listening to the temporomandibular joint. (b) Stereo-stethoscope in use allowing auscultation and comparison of one TMJ with the other. (M. Ziad Al-Ani, Robin J.M. Gray.)

Dental sensitivity is a common symptom of active bruxism. The anterior teeth are often affected and this is frequently noticed on waking from sleep. Repeated tooth and/or restoration fracture is often also reported.

The two most reliable signs of **active** bruxism are, however, scalloping of the lateral border of the tongue (Figure 3.12b) and ridging of the buccal cheek mucosa along the occlusal line (Figure 3.12c). These features are due to the soft tissues being thrust against the surfaces of the teeth during parafunction. Ridging of the cheek mucosa is occasionally severe enough to present clinically as frictional hyperkeratosis. Both scalloping

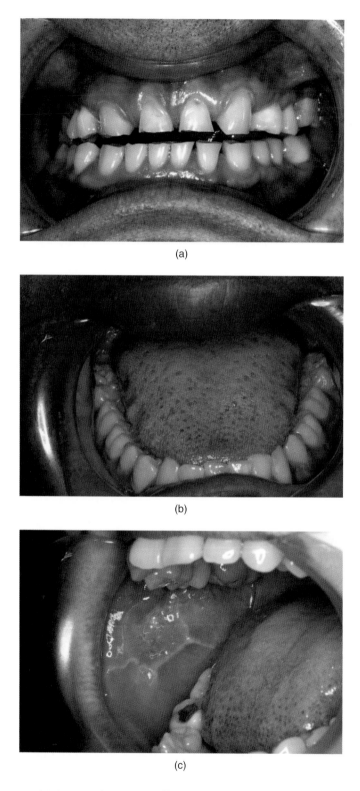

Figure 3.12 (a) Attrition, (b) tongue scalloping, and (c) cheek ridging seen in patients who parafunction. (M. Ziad Al-Ani, Robin J.M. Gray.)

of the tongue and ridging of the cheek mucosa usually disappear when the parafunction ceases.

Occlusal examination 1

For the purposes of occlusal examination of a patient with a TMD, a straightforward examination technique can be employed. Further and more detailed examination will be necessary if it is determined that the occlusion is a major aetiological factor in the TMD or if restorative treatment is planned.

Centric occlusion and centric jaw relation

It is important to determine whether centric occlusion (the habitual bite) coincides with centric jaw relation (the patient's relaxed mandibular position). If these two jaw positions do not coincide (Figure 3.13), it is important to determine where the premature occlusal contact occurs at first tooth contact and what is the direction of the slide from the initial centric relation contact to the patient's habitual bite. If there is premature contact and a small slide from centric relation to centric occlusion, and if in the same sagittal plane, this is not thought to be as clinically significant as a marked lateral slide. The direction and magnitude of the slide are therefore important.

Manipulation of the mandible to centric relation is a difficult technique to master because only very gentle pressure should be applied (Figure 3.14).

The objective is not for the clinician to override the patient's muscle force with his or her own. If manipulation to centric jaw relation is difficult, it is sometimes useful to put a small amount of softened green-stick compound between the upper and lower incisor teeth and help the patient to gently tap into this. This often relaxes the muscles to a degree whereby passive manipulation of the mandible can be achieved. When performing this manoeuvre, it is useful to use thin articulating paper (Baush Occlusion Paper 40 μm) supported in paper holding forceps (Figure 3.15).

The first tooth contact is recorded using the articulating paper and the patient is then requested to squeeze the teeth together and any slide from centric jaw relation to centric occlusion is observed and recorded.

Anterior guidance

To examine all lateral excursions, patients are instructed to close lightly into centric occlusion and subsequently slowly execute maximum active right, left, and protrusive mandibular movements while maintaining contact between the mandibular and maxillary teeth (Figure 3.16).

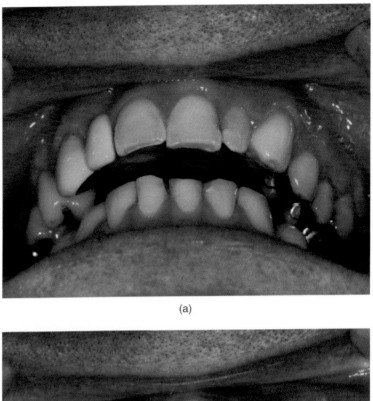

(a)

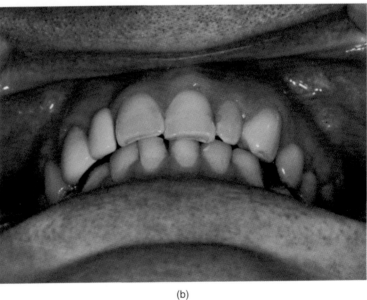

(b)

Figure 3.13 The difference between (a) centric relation and (b) centric occlusion (From Gray RJ, Davies SJ, Quayle AA. A clinical approach to temporomandibular disorders. 4. Examination of the articulatory system: the Occlusion. Br Dent J 1994;177:63–68.)

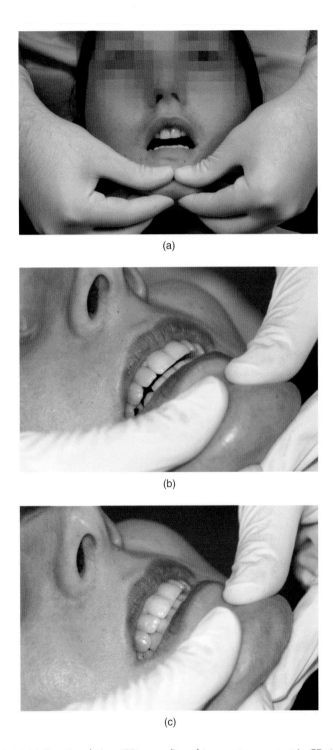

(a)

(b)

(c)

Figure 3.14 (a) Centric relation (CR) recording; (b) premature contact in CR. (c) Slide from CR to centric occlusion observed and recorded. (M. Ziad Al-Ani, Robin J.M. Gray.)

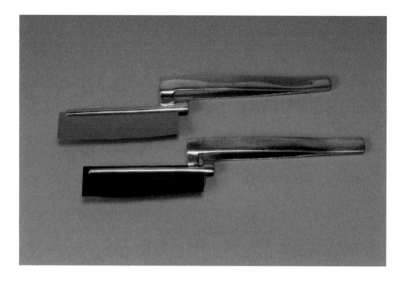

Figure 3.15 Paper-holding forceps: blue for static occlusion; red for dynamic movements. (M. Ziad Al-Ani, Robin J.M. Gray.)

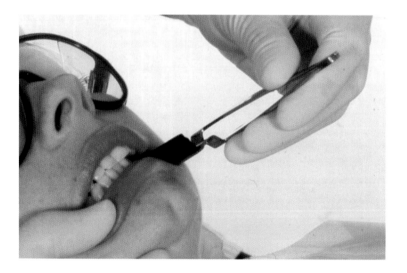

Figure 3.16 Determination of anterior guidance. (M. Ziad Al-Ani, Robin J.M. Gray.)

The anterior guidance in the mandible can be on the canine teeth, which is ideal because this means that the patient can move the mandible from side to side with immediate disclusion of the posterior teeth (Figure 3.17).

There can be group function where the canine, premolar, and molar teeth all contact during lateral excursion of the mandible. This is equally acceptable, preferably with the anterior contact being firmer than the posterior contact.

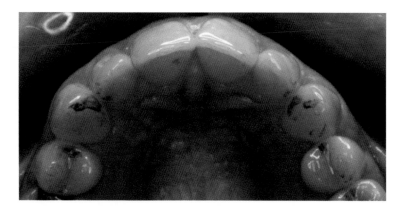

Figure 3.17 Canine guidance. (M. Ziad Al-Ani, Robin J.M. Gray.)

Posterior interferences

If posterior teeth 'get in the way' (interfere), this can be detected by immediate separation of the anterior teeth and guidance of the mandible is then transferred to the interfering tooth. It is thought that interferences, usually on the non-working side (Figure 3.18a) but also on the working side (Figure 3.18b), can be responsible for initiating parafunction. Check for the presence of interferences up to maximum lateral excursions. Patients may parafunction with the mandible in very unlikely and extreme lateral positions, and this may not be clinically evident unless you are meticulous with your examination.

Freedom in centric occlusion

Check whether or not the patient has freedom to move the mandible back and forward with the teeth in light contact when in centric occlusion.

Temporomandibular disorders can be initiated by restorative dental treatment. One situation is for a patient to have anterior crowns placed when he or she has a very tight anterior occlusion such as seen in a patient with an Angle's class II, division II, basal bone and incisal relationship. If crowns are placed on the upper anterior teeth, which are even marginally thicker palatally than the natural teeth were, the effect is to push the mandible distally, thereby compressing the sensitive posterior bilaminar zone of the disc and producing, sometimes severe, pain.

Record-keeping

It is important not only for clinical reasons but also for medicolegal reasons to keep accurate and contemporaneous notes of all aspects of your clinical examinations. Remember that it may be several months or even years later when you might be asked to produce them.

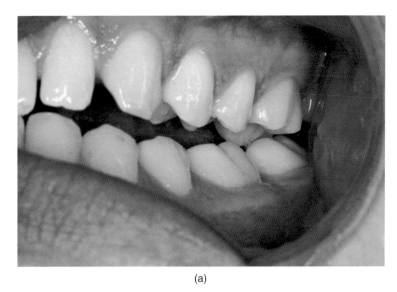

(a)

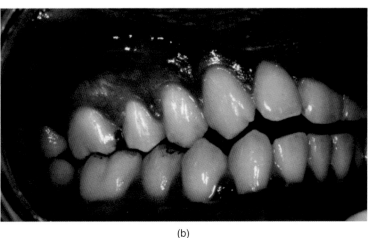

(b)

Figure 3.18 (a) Non-working side interference; (b) working side interference. (From Gray RJ, Davies SJ, Quayle AA. A clinical approach to temporomandibular disorders. 4. Examination of the articulatory system: the Occlusion. Br Dent J 1994;177:63–68.)

Further Reading

Al-Ani, M.Z. and Gray, R.J. (2004). Evaluation of three devices used for measuring mouth opening. *Dent Update* 31: 346–348. 50.

Davies, S.J. and Gray, R.J.M. (2001). The examination and recording of the occlusion: why and how. *Br Dent J* 191: 291–296. 299–302.

Gallagher, C., Gallagher, V., Whelton, H., and Cronin, M. (2004). The normal range of mouth opening in an Irish population. *J Oral Rehabil* 31: 110–116.

Gray, R. and Al-Ani, Z. (2010). Risk management in clinical practice. Part 8. Temporomandibular disorders. *Br Dent J* 209: 433–449.

Gray, R. and Al-Ani, Z. (2013). Conservative temporomandibular disorder management: what DO I do? – frequently asked questions. *Dental Update* 40: 745–756.

Gray, R.J., Davies, S.J., and Quayle, A.A. (1994). A clinical approach to temporomandibular disorders. 2. Examination of the articulatory system: the temporomandibular joints. *Br Dent J* 176: 473–477.

Gray, R.J., Davies, S.J., and Quayle, A.A. (1994). A clinical approach to temporomandibular disorders. 3. Examination of the articulatory system: the muscles. *Br Dent J* 177: 25–28.

Gray, R.J., Davies, S.J., and Quayle, A.A. (1994). A clinical approach to temporomandibular disorders. 4. Examination of the articulatory system: occlusion. *Br Dent J* 177: 63–68.

Gray, R.J., Davies, S.J., and Quayle, A.A. (1994). A clinical approach to temporomandibular disorders. 5. A clinical approach to treatment. *Br Dent J* 177: 101–106.

Juniper, R.P. (1984). Temporomandibular joint dysfunction: a theory based upon electromyographic studies of the lateral pterygoid muscle. *Br J Oral Maxillofac Surg* 22: 18.

Klineberg, I. and Jagger, R. (2004). *Occlusion and Clinical Practice: An Evidence-Based Approach*. London: Wright.

Turp, J.C. and Minagi, S. (2001). Palpation of the lateral pterygoid region in TMD – where is the evidence? *J Dent* 29: 475–483.

Wilson, P.H. and Banerjee, A. (2004). Recording the retruded contact position: a review of clinical techniques. *Br Dent J* 196: 395–402. quiz 426.

Chapter 4

I've Got 'TMJ'!

History

You are confronted in your surgery one morning by a relatively new patient, Mrs Davies, who is a mother of two young children and is a teacher at a nearby private secondary school. On previous examinations, although she has always been polite and friendly, she has insisted on being seen on time and does not like to be kept waiting. She obviously has a very pressurised life that she balances between work and family commitments.

'I have got "TMJ". I have researched it on the internet and I know what needs to be done!' This was her opening comment. She then delivered a rapid synopsis of her symptoms.

You insisted on taking a full and comprehensive history. For the last three weeks, she has woken with pain on the left side of her face. This seems to be centred around her left ear, but extends up into her left temple and down the left mandible into her neck. She said that this side of her face feels 'heavy'. When she wakes in the morning, her jaw feels stiff to move. She complains that her front teeth, especially on the left side, feel generally sensitive. She notices this when she has cold milk on her cereal in the morning, but she said that this gradually wears off as the morning progresses. The teeth were not tender to bite on. After the onset of her symptoms, she went to see her doctor because she thought that she had an ear infection. Her doctor examined her and, although there was no obvious evidence of an ear infection, prescribed some antibiotics. These produced no benefit. She described her discomfort as being a 'dull ache'. She could not put one finger on the main source of her discomfort, indicating rather that it was diffuse. Her symptoms arose gradually and, as far as she was aware, there had been no particular initiating event.

You questioned her about her reduced range of movement and she said that the stiffness in her jaw was there for only a short period in the

Temporomandibular Disorders: A Problem-Based Approach, Second Edition. M. Ziad Al-Ani and Robin J.M. Gray.
© 2021 M. Ziad Al-Ani and Robin J.M. Gray. Published 2021 by John Wiley & Sons Ltd.
Companion Website: www.wiley.com/go/al-ani/temporomandibular-disorders-2e

morning and generally wore off within an hour or so of waking. The limited movement was because of discomfort rather than because of a physical restriction of movement.

You asked her about joint sounds such as jaw joint clicking and she remembered that she had had an intermittent click from her left TMJ a couple of weeks ago but this had disappeared. She did recollect that it may have happened on one or two occasions since then but she could not be sure.

At this point, before you had even had time to start your clinical examination, she said 'Will you X-ray it? I don't want medication but I need a splint!'

On questioning her further, she volunteered that she had researched this topic thoroughly on the Internet and realised that provision of antidepressant medication was quite commonplace in the management of patients with 'TMJ'. She had also read about cranial osteopathy which she thought might help but, most importantly, she knew that her bite could be the cause of the problem because she felt that she had started to grind her teeth.

She wanted you to adjust her bite to stop her doing this and thought that this could also be involved with the headaches that she had been having. She introduced this as a new symptom unrelated to anything that she had talked about previously. When you questioned this she said that she had recently started suffering from a chronic daily headache that was there when she woke in the morning and gradually wore off as the day progressed.

You are therefore left with a confused and confusing story.

Medical history

 Mrs Davies has a history of peptic ulceration and is currently taking cimetidine.

Examination

She had an Angle's class I, basal bone and incisal relationship.

Range of movement

On examination, her range of movement was entirely within normal limits. She could open comfortably to 35 mm, and thereafter to a maximum of 40 mm. She could move her mandible laterally 8 mm to both the right and the left sides. The extreme ranges of movement were not painful but were 'uncomfortable'. When you examined the pathway of her mouth opening, it was straight in the vertical plane. There were no transient or lasting deviations in her mouth movements.

Joint sounds

You listened to her TMJs for joint sounds. There was no evidence of clicking from either the right or the left side on vertical or lateral movement. There was no evidence of any crepitation from either the right or the left side.

Signs of bruxism

You examined her mouth intraorally for signs of active bruxism. She had marked ridging on the inside of her left cheek and generalised scalloping of the lateral border of her tongue on both sides. There was no obvious tooth attrition that could be attributed to parafunction. She did, however, have some occlusal facets that you thought were attributable to normal occlusal wear.

Temporomandibular joint tenderness 2 3

The left TMJ was tender on intra-auricular palpation of the posterior part of the condyle via the external auditory meatus. There was no lateral tenderness on palpation of the preauricular region and no tenderness of the left TMJ on gentle manipulation of the mandible to a retruded position.

Mandibular muscle tenderness 2

On examination of the mandibular muscles, the origin of the left masseter muscle was tender on bimanual palpation along the zygoma, as was the origin of the left temporalis muscle on digital examination in the anterior temporal fossa. There was no particular discomfort elicited on examination of the pterygoid muscles against resistance. There was, however, tenderness of the posterior belly of the digastric muscle on the left side, on palpation behind the ascending ramus of the mandible on the left.

Examination of the muscles on the right side was entirely normal. When you assessed the degree of tenderness of the muscles on the left side, the left temporalis muscle was more tender than the left masseter muscle.

Occlusion 1

On examination of her occlusion, centric jaw relation and centric occlusion did not coincide. There was a premature contact in centric jaw relation between the upper and lower first molars on the left side, and an obvious but small vertical and left slide from centric relation to centric occlusion when she was asked to squeeze her teeth together.

When you examined excursive movements of her mandible, there was interference on the non-working side between the upper and lower left first molars on right lateral mandibular excursion. There were no obvious interferences on the working side of either side and those on the non-working side did not extend beyond the canine crossover position. There was freedom in centric occlusion.

Intraoral examination

When you considered her general dental health she had good oral hygiene, there were no plaque or calculus deposits. She had a basic periodontal examination (BPE) of one in each sextant and minimal occlusal restorations. There was no active caries or periodontal disease. She was a regular six-monthly dental attender.

Special tests

Although she requested a radiograph, you did not feel that it was justified to take radiographs of either her teeth or her TMJs. She had recently had bite-wing radiographs taken which showed there to be no deficient restorations or active caries and you could not see the justification for exposing her to radiation by radiographic examination of the TMJs because you could see no clinical need for doing so – Ionising Radiations (Medical Exposure) Regulations (IR(ME)R) 2018.

Differential diagnosis

Always consider all your options – keep an open mind.

Mrs Davies was adamant that she had 'TMJ'. It is important not to be swayed by a patient's perceived wisdom from unreliable sources (the internet). You must always base your diagnosis and treatment plan on evidence-based knowledge. The clinical position of the dentist is to analyse the symptoms and come to his or her own conclusion, no matter how much pressure he or she may be put under by the patient. The provisional diagnosis in this case is fairly straightforward. There is no indication of active dental disease of any form. She did complain of headache, but this was a secondary complaint, and that she said was related to her problems from her jaw. She did not describe her headache as being her primary complaint. She also said that she had had clicking from her jaw joint but again remembered this only on prompting as being an occasional complaint and was of secondary clinical significance.

She thought that she had started a parafunctional activity such as bruxism or clenching but said that she was now unsure of this because her husband had never heard her grind her teeth in her sleep. Patients can, however, grind or clench their teeth without producing noise. You must not dismiss the possibility of parafunctional habits just because their sleeping partner has not heard them. A diagnosis of this being an ENT problem had been excluded by her doctor and antibiotics had not altered her symptoms in any way.

Final diagnosis for Mrs Davies

Myofascial pain (facial arthromyalgia; pain dysfunction syndrome).

Management

Explanation and reassurance

You may be faced with a patient such as Mrs Davies who has researched her symptoms on the Internet and comes to you with several convictions that are perceived wisdom or half-truths, or that may or may not be correct. It is important for you at this stage to take the lead and establish and agree with her what is and what is not accurate. Explain that the correct term for her condition is a 'TMD' not a 'TMJ' because the joint is only one component of the articulatory system, and the muscles and occlusion may also be involved.

Explanation of parafunctional activity is important. Patients will often deny that they perform such an activity even though they have clinical signs of active bruxism, such as cheek ridging or tongue scalloping. In addition, if the teeth are often sensitive on waking they are usually more ready to accept that such a feature does exist.

Physiotherapy

Myofascial pain is a musculoskeletal disorder and physiotherapy plays a major role in its management. Physiotherapy can take the form of electrophysiotherapy such as megapulse (Figure 4.1), ultrasound (Figure 4.2), soft laser (Figure 4.3), acupuncture (Figure 4.4), or manipulation of the muscles and mobilisation of the joints.

Any modality that a physiotherapist recommends is acceptable in a patient with myofascial pain as long as there is no risk of damage to the intrajoint structures and treatment does not worsen other symptoms. Forced attempts to improve mouth opening are to be avoided. Leave the choice of therapy to the physiotherapist.

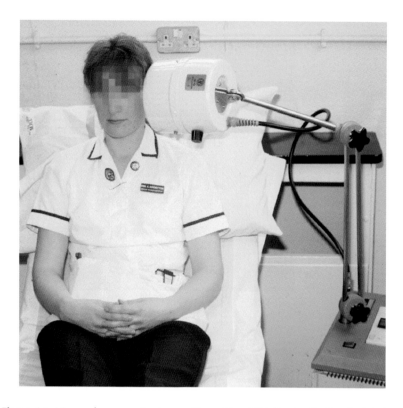

Figure 4.1 Megapulse apparatus in use. (From Gray RJM, Davies SJ, Quayle AA. A clinical approach to temporomandibular disorders. 5. A clinical approach to treatment. Br Dent J 1994;177:101–106 with permission.)

Soft laser

The results of a recent meta-analysis of randomized controlled trials of the efficacy of low-level laser therapy in the treatment of TMDs have provided the best evidence in this regard. This study indicated that using low-level laser therapy has limited efficacy in reducing pain in patients with TMDs but it can significantly improve the functional outcomes of patients with TMDs. The most commonly used wavelength is located in the electromagnetic spectrum from 780 to 904 nm.

Acupuncture

Is there any evidence to support the use of acupuncture in TMD management?

It is claimed that acupuncture has a beneficial role in TMD management, principally of myofacial pain, and that the use of acupuncture has a success rate similar to that of occlusal splints and other treatments in relieving symptoms.

A systematic review of the literature has been conducted to determine the effectiveness of acupuncture in treating myofascial pain and concluded that despite the weak scientific supporting its efficacy,

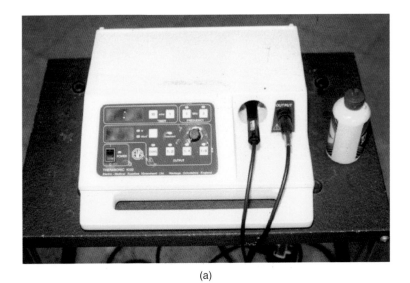

(a)

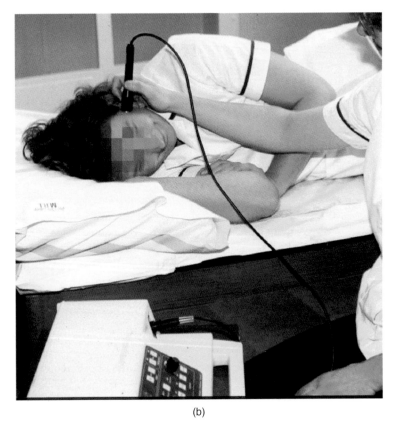

(b)

Figure 4.2 (a) Ultrasound apparatus; (b) ultrasound apparatus in use. (Gray RJM, Davies SJ, Quayle AA. A clinical approach to temporomandibular disorders. 5. A clinical approach to treatment. Br Dent J 1994;177:101–106 with permission.)

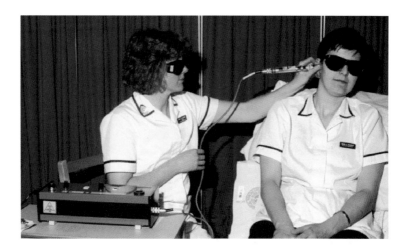

Figure 4.3 Soft laser apparatus in use. (M. Ziad Al-Ani, Robin J.M. Gray.)

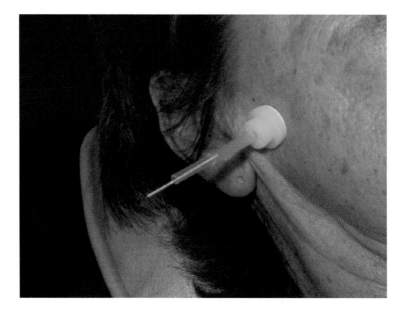

Figure 4.4 Acupuncture in the management of myofascial pain. (M. Ziad Al-Ani, Robin J.M. Gray.)

acupuncture treatment appears to relieve signs and symptoms of pain in myofascial TMD.

A recent randomized controlled trial found a significant but non-specific reduction in pain among patients with non-chronic painful TMD after four weeks of acupuncture treatment, and it concluded that acupuncture should be considered as a first-line treatment option, preferably in combination with other treatments.

However, owing to several methodological flaws, evidence remains inconclusive and the efficacy of acupuncture cannot be ascertained based on current literature.

Drug therapy

In cases of acute pterygoid muscle spasm associated with disc displacement with reduction, Temazepam as Temazepam Oral Suspension, can be prescribed. Benzodiazepines have a pharmacologically recognised muscle relaxant effect. This would not be appropriate in this case because the lateral pterygoid muscle was not tender. Non-steroidal anti-inflammatory drugs (NSAIDs) can be used but should be strictly avoided when there is any history of gastric irritation. Remember that this patient was on medication for peptic ulceration.

Splint therapy 7

Mrs Davies had downloaded a page from an article that she had found on the Internet describing the design of splint that she wanted. The photograph showed a partial coverage splint fitted to the lower arch, with acrylic covering the occlusal surfaces of the molar and premolar teeth on both the right and the left sides connected by a stainless steel lingual bar (Figure 4.5).

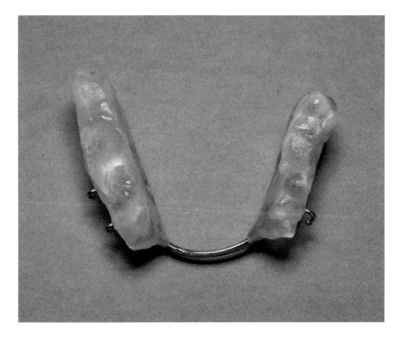

Figure 4.5 Photograph of a partial coverage splint brought by patient. (M. Ziad Al-Ani, Robin J.M. Gray.)

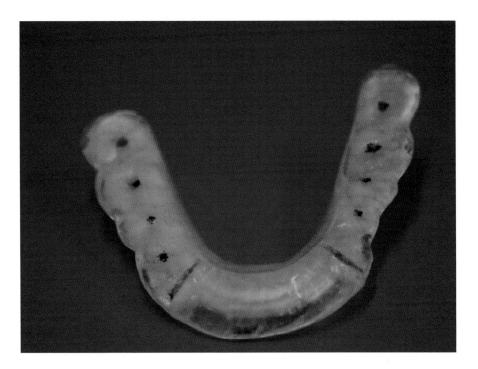

Figure 4.6 A balanced stabilisation splint: blue, static; red, dynamic occlusal contacts. (M. Ziad Al-Ani, Robin J.M. Gray.)

She said that she would be happy to wear this all day and night if necessary because it would not be obvious and socially embarrassing and her school class might not notice.

 You explain the rationale behind your decision not to construct such an appliance and suggest that the splint of choice would be an occlusally balanced stabilisation splint (Figure 4.6).

You should also explain your reasons for your decision in prescribing this appliance in relation to her parafunctional habit because it will provide her with an improved occlusion when she wears it and will lead to muscle relaxation. You must be adamant that partial coverage splints should be avoided because they cause occlusal disruption.

You did discuss provision of an occlusal interference splint with her but, when you examined the wear facets on her teeth, it was apparent that her bruxism was in a lateral excursion so this would render this simpler design of splint ineffective.

With proper clinical examination and explanation of the perceived mode of action of splint therapy, the dangers of inappropriate treatment and the rationale for outpatient physiotherapy, your treatment plan was accepted, treatment proceeded uneventfully, and her symptoms resolved.

After wearing the splint for just over three months, a successful weaning-off period took place and she now wears the splint on only an 'as-needed' basis.

Further Reading

Carraro, J.J. and Caffesse, R.G. (1978). Effect of occlusal splints on TMJ symptomatology. *J Prosthet Dent* 40: 563–566.

Clark, G.T. (1984). A critical evaluation of orthopaedic interocclusal appliance therapy. Design, theory, and overall effectiveness. *J Am Dent Assoc* 108: 359–365.

Davies, S.J. and Gray, R.J.M. (1997). The pattern of splint usage in the management of two common temporomandibular disorders. Part III: Long-term follow-up in an assessment of splint therapy in the management of disc displacement with reduction and pain dysfunction syndrome. *Br Dent J* 183: 279–283.

Gray, R.J.M. and Davies, S.J. (2001). Occlusal splints and temporomandibular disorders: why, when, how? *Dent Update* 28: 194–199.

Gray, R.J.M., Davies, S.J., and Quayle, A.A. (1991). A comparison of two splints in the treatment of TMJ pain dysfunction syndrome. Can occlusal analysis be used to predict success of splint therapy? *Br Dent J* 170: 55–58.

Gray, R.J.M., Davies, S.J., and Quayle, A.A. (1994). A clinical approach to temporomandibular disorders. 5.A clinical approach to treatment. *Br Dent J* 177: 101–106.

Kurita, H., Kurashina, K., and Kotani, A. (1997). Clinical effect of full coverage occlusal splint therapy for specific temporomandibular disorder conditions and symptoms. *J Prosthet Dent* 78: 506–510.

Lobbezoo, F. and Naeije, M. (2001). Bruxism is mainly regulated centrally, not peripherally: review. *J Oral Rehabil* 28: 1085–1091.

Lobbezoo, F. and Lavigne, G.J. (1997). Do bruxism and temporomandibular disorders have a cause-and-effect relationship? *J Orofac Pain* 11: 15–23.

Manfredini, D., Bucci, M.B., Sabattini, V.B., and Lobbezoo, F. (2011). Bruxism: overview of current knowledge and suggestions for dental implants planning. *Cranio* 29: 304–312.

Simma, I., Gleditsch, J.M., Simma, L., and Piehslinger, E. (2009). Immediate effects of microsystem acupuncture in patients with oromyofacial pain and craniomandibular disorders (CMD): a double-blind, placebo-controlled trial. *Br Dent J* 12: E26.

Shimada, A., Ishigaki, S., Matsuka, Y. et al. (2019). Effects of exercise therapy on painful temporomandibular disorders. *J Oral Rehabil* 46: 475–481.

Talaat, A.M., el-Dibany, M.M., and el-Garf, A. (1986). Physical therapy in the management of myofascial pain dysfunction syndrome. *Ann Otol Rhinol Laryngol* 95: 225–228.

Wassell, R.W., Adams, N., and Kelly, P.J. (2004). Treatment of temporomandibular disorders by stabilising splints in general dental practice: results after initial treatment. *Br Dent J* 197: 35–41. discussion 31; quiz 50–1.

Wassell, R.W., Adams, N., and Kelly, P.J. (2006). The treatment of temporomandibular disorders with stabilizing splints in general dental practice: one-year follow-up. *J Am Dent Assoc* 137: 1089–1098. quiz 1168–9.

Evidence-based Dentistry

Al-Ani, M.Z., Davies, S.J., Gray, R.J.M. et al. (2004). Does splint therapy work for temporomandibular pain? *Evidence-Based Dent* 5: 65–66.

Chen, J., Huang, Z., Ge, M., and Gao, M. (2015). Efficacy of low-level laser therapy in the treatment of TMD s: a meta-analysis of 14 randomised controlled trials. *J Oral Rehabil* 42: 291–299.

Fernandes, A.C., Duarte Moura, D.M., Da Silva, L.G.D. et al. (2017). Acupuncture in temporomandibular disorder myofascial pain treatment: a systematic review. *J Oral Facial Pain Headache* 31 (3): 225–232.

Macedo, C.R., Silva, A.B., Machado, M.A. et al. (2008). The effectiveness of occlusal splints for sleep bruxism. *Evidence-Based Dent* 9: 23.

Munguia, F.M., Jang, J., Salem, M. et al. (2018). Efficacy of low-level laser therapy in the treatment of temporomandibular myofascial pain: a systematic review and meta-analysis. *J Oral Facial Pain Headache* 32 (3): 287–297.

Şen, S., Orhan, G., Sertel, S. et al. (2020). Comparison of acupuncture on specific and non-specific points for the treatment of painful temporomandibular disorders: a randomised controlled trial. *J Oral Rehabil* 47: 783–795.

Smith, P., Mosscrop, D., Davies, S. et al. (2007). The efficacy of acupuncture in the treatment of ftemporomandibular joint myofascial pain: a randomized controlled trial. *J Dent* 35: 259–267.

Chapter 5

I've Got a Clicking Joint

History

Mrs Smith is a 30-year-old woman who complains of occasionally painful clicking from her right temporomandibular joint (TMJ).

The history of her present complaint is that a painless click had been present for 14 years. This arose with sudden onset and no initiating event. Ever since she has had consistent clicking from the right TMJ which never comes and goes but does vary in intensity. She has never experienced locking. The clicking is worse (louder) with function, as in when eating. Originally, it was not present when she talked but now it is. She reported that the click was worse in the morning when she woke up and her jaw felt stiff. This stiffness was present for only an hour or so and then her movement returned to normal. The click, however, remained.

More recently the click has become 'uncomfortable' and she said that her bite now 'feels odd'. She has noticed that, when she stands in front of a mirror and opens her mouth, her jaw does not move in a straight line.

Mrs Smith attended her general medical practitioner who suggested referral for a dental opinion.

She has no medical history of note and is not taking any medication. She was a fit and healthy person. She had, however, been stressed at work over the last two years because she was worried about possible redundancy. She is a secretary and spends a lot of time on the telephone and now finds her click embarrassing because it has occasionally started to happen while talking and customers have questioned her about it.

Temporomandibular Disorders: A Problem-Based Approach, Second Edition. M. Ziad Al-Ani and Robin J.M. Gray.
© 2021 M. Ziad Al-Ani and Robin J.M. Gray. Published 2021 by John Wiley & Sons Ltd.
Companion Website: www.wiley.com/go/al-ani/temporomandibular-disorders-2e

Examination 1

She has a class I, basal bone and incisal relationship.

She can open to well within the normal range (40 mm) in the vertical dimension. She can move equally easily to both the right and the left sides to over 10 mm. There is no discomfort on vertical or lateral jaw movements.

She has a transient deviation when examining the pathway of opening. Her mouth deviates to the right when opening wide, but after this deviation the pathway of opening returns to the vertical.

She has a midcycle reciprocal (opening and closing) click from the right TMJ. The opening click is audible to others and is louder than the closing click which could be heard only with the use of a stethoscope.

On intraoral examination, there was ridging of the buccal mucosa and abnormal attrition of her teeth, especially the upper and lower left and right canines, and the buccal cusp tip of the lower left second premolar and first molar.

The temporalis and masseter muscles were examined by palpation and the lateral pterygoid against resistance. There were no obvious areas of muscle tenderness but opening against resistance was 'uncomfortable'. She said that her face had on occasion been aching when she wakes in the morning, as it had today.

The TMJs were examined by direct palpation in the preauricular region and via the external auditory meatus. There was no evidence of TMJ tenderness on lateral palpation but the right TMJ was tender when examined via the external auditory meatus with her mouth both open and closed.

On examination of the occlusion, she appeared to have centric relation occlusion; there were no premature contacts and no slide from centric relation to centric occlusion. She had canine guidance on both the right and the left sides. There were interferences on the working side involving the right premolars and first molar, and there were interferences on the non-working side involving the upper and lower left molars.

Radiographs

These are not usually relevant. A radiograph should be taken only if it is essential for the dentist to reach a diagnosis or if the treatment plan depends upon the outcome of it. In this instance, the clinician would expect the radiograph to be perfectly normal, because it is the soft tissues of the TMJ that are involved.

The normal radiographs used to visualise the TMJ are a dental panoramic tomogram (DPT) (Figure 5.1), or a transpharyngeal (Figure 5.2) or transcranial oblique lateral (TOL) view of the skull (Figure 5.3).

As both the articulating surfaces of the joint and the disc are fibrous tissue, these components cannot be visualised on a radiograph. Only a small portion of the articulating surface is visible and, especially with

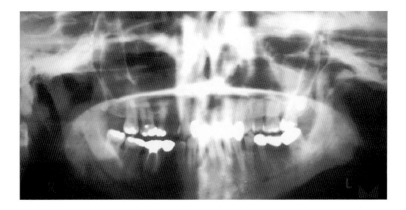

Figure 5.1 Dental panoramic tomographs used to show condyles. (M. Ziad Al-Ani, Robin J.M. Gray.)

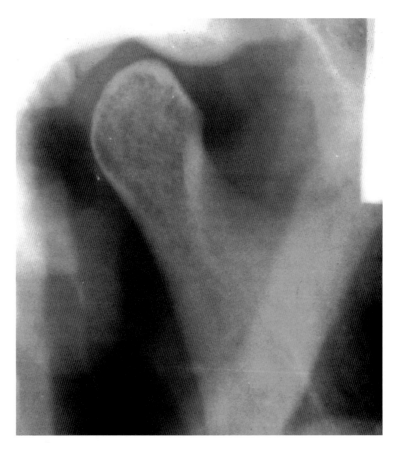

Figure 5.2 Transpharyngeal view of the mandibular condyle. (M. Ziad Al-Ani, Robin J.M. Gray.)

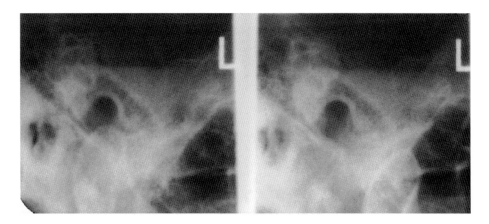

Figure 5.3 Transcranial oblique lateral radiographs. (M. Ziad Al-Ani, Robin J.M. Gray.)

the TOL, the articulating surfaces shown are not load-bearing parts of the joint. There must be approximately 40% decalcification before bony erosions can be visualised. The joint space cannot be estimated, and the position of the disc cannot be identified.

For all these reasons, radiographs of TMJs are of limited value, as are other scanning methods unless invasive treatment is being planned.

According to (IR(ME)R) 2018 guidelines, it is your responsibility to minimise the radiation exposure for patients and radiographs should be taken only when clinically essential.

Other special tests

In this lady's case, the click disappeared on anterior posturing of the mandible.

When she opened and closed her mouth from her habitual bite, the click was consistently present. It was louder on opening and softer on closing but was present on every opening and closing cycle. When she postured her mandible forwards until the incisors were in an edge-to-edge relationship, and opened and closed from this protrusive position, the click disappeared after the first opening cycle.

Why do TMJs click?   (S)4

First think about the anatomy of the joint.

The components of the TMJ involve the fossa in the petrous part of the temporal bone and the condylar process of the mandible. Interposed between the two bony components is the intra-articular disc which is a sheet of fibrous tissue. It has attachments circumferentially around the head of the condyle. There is an elastic attachment to the area of the squamotympanic fissure on the base of the skull, and a fibrous attachment to the posterior part of the neck of the condyle. Anteriorly the disc is confluent with and inserts into the superior pterygoid muscle (superior head of the lateral pterygoid muscle).

The disc is divided into three zones: a thick posterior band, a thin intermediate zone, and a slightly thicker but narrow anterior band. The shape of the disc is described as being similar to a 'jockey's cap', with the peak anteriorly in the region of the pterygoid muscle attachment (Chapter 2). This disc therefore divides the joint capsule into two spaces: the superior and the inferior joint spaces. The inferior joint space is between the underside of the surface of the disc and the head of the condyle. The superior joint space is between the superior surface of the disc and the articular fossa.

During the first phase of mouth opening, condylar movement in the joint capsule is purely rotational and occurs in the inferior joint space. The first part of mouth opening is principally a 'hinge' action and rotation occurs between the head of the condyle and the inferior surface of the disc. The amount of mouth opening that can be attained during this phase is remarkably consistent and is between 17 and 20 mm.

The second phase of joint movement is a translational or sliding movement which occurs mainly in the superior joint cavity. During this phase of movement, the head of the condyle moves forwards from resting against the posterior band of the disc, slides over the intermediate zone, and finally on to the anterior band of the disc as the whole complex slides down the anterior slope of the articular eminence.

The disc is pulled forward by the superior head of the lateral pterygoid muscle and the posterior attachment to the squamotympanic fissure, which is elastic, allows stretching of this portion of the disc, thereby allowing it to remain interposed between the two bony components of the joint at all phases of movement. During closure of the mouth, the reverse process occurs and the elastic recoil of the posterior part of the bilaminar zone of the disc helps to pull it back into place (Figure 5.4).

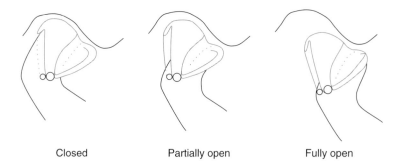

| Closed | Partially open | Fully open |

Figure 5.4 Normal condyle disc fossa relationship during mouth opening. (Davies SJ, Gray RJM.1997, The pattern of splint usage in the management of two common temporomandibular disorders. Part I: The anterior repositioning splint in the treatment of disc displacement with reduction. Br Dent J; 183:199–203.© 1997, Spring Nature.)

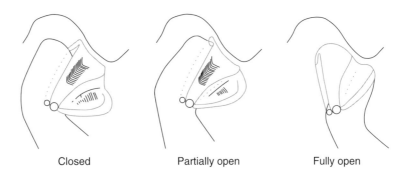

Closed   Partially open   Fully open

Figure 5.5 Anteriorly displaced reducing disc in relation to condyle during mouth opening. (Davies SJ, Gray RJM.1997, The pattern of splint usage in the management of two common temporomandibular disorders. Part I: The anterior repositioning splint in the treatment of disc displacement with reduction. Br Dent J; 183:199–203.© 1997, Spring Nature.)

If the joint is damaged or overloaded in any way, there is a tendency for an increased tonicity in the pterygoid muscle and this tends to pull the disc forwards. The rotational phase of mouth opening still occurs as normal, but as the translation phase starts, the head of the condyle slides forwards and encounters the disc in the displaced position and it impacts against the thicker posterior band of the disc. Friction is then built up until the head of the condyle 'jumps past' this portion of the disc which causes an audible release of energy, which is the click (Figure 5.5).

The click appears to be the sound produced by the sudden distraction of the opposing wet surfaces of the disc and condyle. It has also been proposed that TMJ clicking occurs because an abnormal relationship between the TMJ components might obstruct the normal movement of the synovial fluid during function, causing fluid to trap under pressure.

The reason that clicking disappears with anterior posturing of the mandible is that bringing the mandible forwards re-establishes a 'normal functional' relationship between the position of the disc and the head of the condyle. This then releases the abnormal fluid pressure that resulted in the click.

When do TMJs click?

 There are two main situations when TMJ clicking occurs. The first is clicking secondary to myofascial pain. This is the click that is present in the patient who may parafunction (clench or grind) during sleep.

In many people who exhibit a parafunctional activity, it is nocturnal and at its most pronounced in the rapid eye movement period of sleep. This is the lighter plane of sleep before waking.

Due to the general increased tonicity in the muscles, there is a tendency for the superior pterygoid muscle to displace the disc anteriorly, which means that there is a click present when the patient wakes up in the morning. As the mandible starts to move during normal function, the increased tone in the pterygoid muscle gradually reverts to normal. This muscle then relaxes, thereby allowing the disc to reposition. The frequent pattern is for there to be a click in the morning on waking for the first hour or so which gradually disappears and is not present during the day, unless at times of increased function, i.e. meal times. This click can sometimes be accompanied by discomfort due to the increased muscle tone and muscle spasm.

Clicking secondary to disc displacement with reduction is altogether a different scenario, and this is what appears to be present with Mrs Smith.

In this situation, the click is initially painless and consistently present, in that it is present on waking but remains during the day and is heard or felt every time the patient opens and closes her mouth beyond a certain point. This click is usually painless until the late stages when discomfort can occur in the posterior bilaminar zone due to the constant stretching of this highly innervated tissue.

This click is described as reciprocal in that it is present during both opening and closing phases of the jaw movement. Opening clicks can be heard more easily and closing clicks less easily. This is because, when the mouth is open, friction builds up displacing the disc until it forcibly repositions with a release of energy. A closing click is, however, more passive because the disc tends merely to fall back into place as the mouth closes.

Early, intermediate and late clicking refer to the stage of mouth opening at which the clicking occurs. Early clicking, which occurs at the start of the opening phase, implies a mild displacement of the disc and, in general, the later in the opening cycle that the click occurs the greater the degree of disc displacement, and the click is usually louder. In addition, clicking can be single or multiple, the latter implying an unstable disc or on occasions an associated perforation or clicking across the different zones of the disc. This is, however, of little clinical importance, apart from perforation, because the treatment methods remain the same.

Why does the mouth deviate when opening?

 The reason why the mouth deviates on opening is that, if there is disc displacement on one side, mandibular opening occurs until the head of the condyle impacts on the displaced disc on the affected side, having an effect on further translation.

The patient may undertake a subconscious deviation of the mandible to 'get past' the disc, after which mouth opening occurs to the normal extent and usually with the midlines coincident. This is what Mrs Smith experiences.

Anterior displacement of the disc with reduction is therefore usually associated with a transient shift of the mandibular midline towards the affected side during mouth opening and sometimes during closing. This is a result of prevention of the normal condylar translation caused by the displaced disc on the affected side, and a resultant transient lateral movement in the opening cycle. The midlines will return to the same vertical plane when the disc condyle relationship normalises after the click.

What preliminary investigations may you use?

 Auscultation, intra- and periauricular palpation and testing the clicking with protrusion of the mandible are all sensible first options.

When the patient postures forwards onto his/her incisor teeth, the head of the condyle projects downwards and forwards so that the displaced disc assumes a more normal 'functional' relationship to the head of the condyle. Opening and closing from this position without causing the click thereby eliminates trauma to the disc and the natural elasticity of the posterior part of the disc gradually repositions it (Figure 5.6).

Radiographs

Not routinely.

MRI, arthography

Not necessary.

Auscultation and intra- and periauricular palpation are simple approaches involving clinical examination and are usually all that is needed to confirm the diagnosis.

Expensive diagnostic measures such as magnetic resonance imaging (MRI) and even arthography should be reserved for surgical planning and, in some cases, to assist diagnosis in more complex pathological conditions of the TMJ. These are not necessary for confirmation of a diagnosis of disc displacement with reduction. A general rule is that any such tests should be used only when they are essential in diagnosis or in determining a treatment plan or will ultimately change the treatment plan.

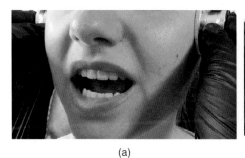   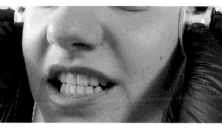

(a)   (b)

Figure 5.6 (a, b) Testing the clicking with protrusion of the mandible. (M. Ziad Al-Ani, Robin J.M. Gray.)

In addition to lateral palpation and intra-auricular palpation of the TMJ via the external auditory meatus, the click from disc displacement with reduction can be detected using a stereo-stethoscope. This consists of standard earpieces with two outlets rather than one and two tubes, each of which is connected to a separate diaphragm. This provides a method of accurately and reproducibly detecting TMJ sounds when trying to determine whether they emanate from the right or the left side or are bilateral. In addition, examination with a stereo-stethoscope allows the clinician to detect a frequently softer closing click which is sometimes not evident or difficult to detect on joint palpation alone.

What is the most likely diagnosis for Mrs Smith?

Clicking secondary to myofascial pain? Possible but unlikely.

Clicking secondary to disc displacement with reduction? Much more likely.

Disc displacement refers to an abnormal relationship at rest and during function of the articular disc to the mandibular condyle and articular eminence. The disc is considered displaced if the inferior concavity of the central intermediate thinner zone of the disc is anterior to the prominence of the condyle. This condition may occur due to injury of the bilaminar zone, the disc or its attachments. Although pathological displacement of the disc can occur in any direction, anterior and anteromedial displacements are the most common.

Why is this? Think about the pull of the lateral pterygoid muscle. This muscle is important in mouth opening and originates from the lateral surface of the lateral pterygoid plate and the infra-temporal surface of the greater wing of the sphenoid; it inserts into the neck of the condyle and the disc, so the pull of this muscle is anteromedial. As the superior head is attached to the disc, if the disc is displaced by increased tone of this muscle, the disc displacement will by its nature also be anteromedial.

Disc displacement with reduction implies that the displaced disc returns to a normal position relative to the condyle on mouth opening. This is characterised by a click that occurs when the condyle slides over the posterior edge of the disc during reduction of the displacement.

The aetiology of disc displacement has not been clearly established because different studies have failed to include specific occlusal, orthodontic, or parafunctional activities as these seem to be equally distributed among people who are and are not patients. The overwhelming majority of patients have no idea what the initiating factor in their symptoms is.

Microtrauma, such as parafunctional activity, or macrotrauma, such as whiplash, external trauma and excessive jaw opening, have been suggested as causative factors of disc displacement.

Hypertonicity in the superior head of the lateral pterygoid muscle has also been suggested as an important aetiological factor causing disc displacement.

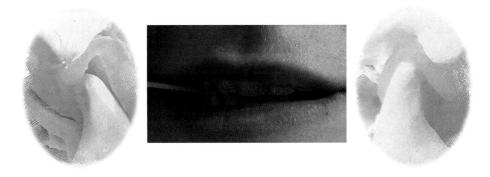

Figure 5.7 Tongue blade test for allocating the source of pain. Biting on a tongue blade on a right side will reduce the pain in the right disc. (M. Ziad Al-Ani, Robin J.M. Gray.)

Is disc displacement painful?

Sometimes, but this depends on the diagnosis.

In general, true internal derangement of disc displacement with reduction is not painful. Pain tends to present in cases of acute disc displacement due to either stretching of the innervated posterior bilaminar zone of the disc or secondary muscle spasm in the later stages of the disorder. The pain associated with acute displacement can be explained by trauma from the condyle against the innervated area of the retrodiscal tissues and capsule, which become non-physiologically stretched. Pain can also be experienced in acute disc displacement when the patient tries to close the molar teeth together and bite down hard. This is often described as a sharp shooting pain.

Think about this! If the disc tissue was well innervated or had a rich blood supply, then every time she clenched her teeth she would compress this tissue and it would be painful. The source of this pain appears to be related to compression of the now stretched, highly innervated, posterior bilaminar zone interposed between the condyle and fossa.

A simple test which can be used to confirm the source of pain in the cases of acute disc displacement is to use the tongue spatula test. Biting on a tongue blade on a right side for example, will reduce the right side pain while biting on the blade on the left side will increase the pain on the right side (Figure 5.7)

How should disc displacement with reduction be managed? Does it always need treatment? Ⓢ5

Sometimes but not always. This depends on the diagnosis and the patient's needs.

Often treatment of painless and otherwise symptomless clicking may be unwarranted due to the patient's lack of concern or unwillingness to wear a splint – the usual method of therapy. Consider also the lack of predictability that the symptom will always resolve with treatment or that it will necessarily create problems in the future.

Treatment of clicking is, however, potentially justified if it becomes a social embarrassment to the patient. It is also prudent to advise treatment of a click if it is associated with pain or locking, either of which may indicate disc instability.

If a patient presents with clicking that has been present for many years and has never caused any other problems whatsoever, there may be no need to treat this condition. The patient may simply be looking for reassurance that it will not deteriorate, cause subsequent arthritic changes to the joint later on, or be due to a possibly sinister cause.

If treatment is indicated, conservative management has been considered adequate for the overwhelming majority of patients with disc displacement.

Treatment

Explanation and reassurance

This demands that you be a sympathetic clinician, have an understandable explanation of the problem, its possible multifactorial aetiology, and the anatomy of the joint and disc, and be able to deliver a carefully explained and justified course of action. It should be explained that some symptoms may persist but equally, in some cases, spontaneous recovery may occur if the symptoms have only recently presented. Reassurance to the patient that this is a common problem and has no sinister cause often helps. Explanation of a hitherto unknown parafunctional habit and dietary advice are also useful and a general advice sheet can be given.

Physiotherapy

Physiotherapy in the acute stage of a disorder, especially if there is associated muscle tenderness as there now seems to be for Mrs Smith, is beneficial and the earlier it is undertaken in the course of the disorder the more beneficial it will be in resolving muscle spasm. If she had not had tenderness, there would be little point in referral at this stage.

Physiotherapy can take many forms but aggressive exercise and effort should be avoided, especially in the case of an acute disc displacement because encouraging the patient to undertake exercises or to stretch opening of the mouth can exacerbate the disc displacement.

Normal methods of electrophysiotherapy usually involve ultrasound or acupuncture, both of which are readily available, or megapulse or soft laser, which are less so.

The frequency of physiotherapy should be a minimum of twice and preferably three times a week for three to four weeks until approximately 10–12 sessions have been delivered. Continued treatment beyond this level should be up to the individual physiotherapist, but there is little evidence to support that ongoing treatment at a lesser frequency will deliver enhanced benefit.

Drug therapy

Prescription of tricyclic antidepressants has little, if any, part to play in the management of chronic disc displacement. Some practitioners feel that prescriptions of a tricyclic antidepressant such as amitriptyline or nortriptyline is of benefit. There is, however, no scientific evidence to substantiate this view.

Prescription of a benzodiazepine, such as Temazepam Oral Suspension, does have a muscle-relaxant role to play in the management of sudden-onset acute disc displacement that causes locking, but does not have a part to play in chronic clicking.

Anterior repositioning splint 7

The anterior repositioning splint (ARPS) is a full-coverage splint constructed on the lower arch, which guides the mandible downwards and forwards into a protrusive position to correct the disc condyle incoordination (Figure 5.8).

The aim of the splint is to place the mandible into a new protrusive position for a therapeutic period of time, usually three months. Maintaining this position can be achieved by the indentations and ramps on the occluding surface of the splint, with which the upper teeth engage; this guides the mandible into a specific protrusive position and allows no

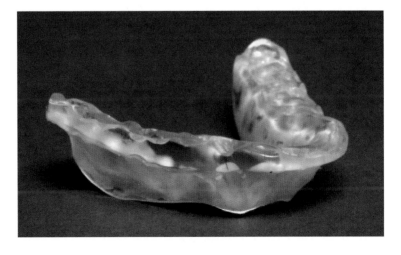

Figure 5.8 Anterior repositioning splint. (M. Ziad Al-Ani, Robin J.M. Gray.)

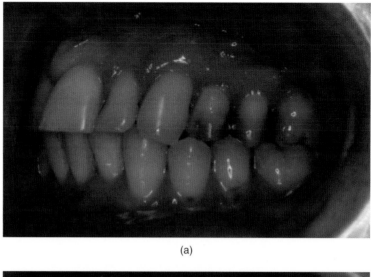

(a)

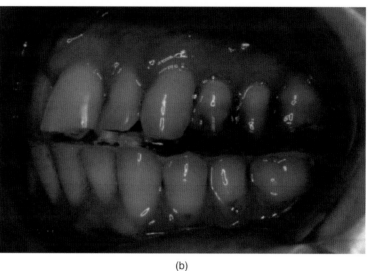

(b)

Figure 5.9 (a) Mandibular position without anterior repositioning splint (ARPS); (b) mandibular position with ARPS. (M. Ziad Al-Ani, Robin J.M. Gray.)

other comfortable position of the mandible on maximum closure against the surface of the appliance (Figure 5.9).

The degree of protrusion is determined at the chair side. It may well be that a patient with an Angle's class II, division I, basal bone, and incisal relationship does not need to come as far forward as incisal edge to edge. If the patient closes in centric occlusion and slowly slides the mandible forwards, the clinician should be able to hear or feel the point at which the click occurs. Immediately, past this degree of protrusion should be the position in which the jaw registration for the appliance is recorded. It is not necessary for the mandible to be positioned any further

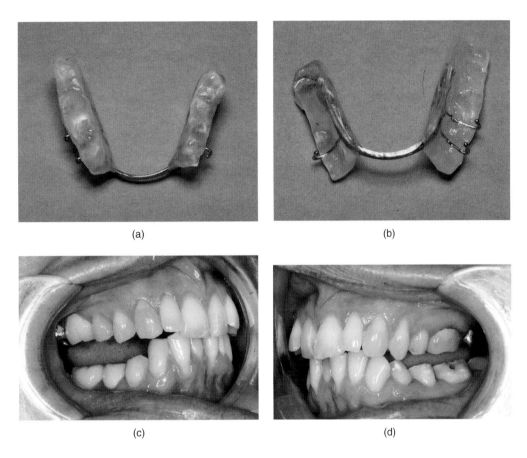

Figure 5.10 (a, b) A partial coverage appliance. (c, d) Disturbed occlusion after treatment with a partial coverage appliance. (M. Ziad Al-Ani, Robin J.M. Gray.)

forward because no additional benefit will be gained. Indeed, the resultant appliance would be very thick and difficult for the patient to tolerate.

It is essential that the splint be full coverage otherwise a partial-coverage appliance will permit unpredictable and unwanted occlusal changes (Figure 5.10). Such appliances are medicolegally indefensible.

The mechanism of this splint is based on the theory that, in patients with disc displacement with reduction, guiding the mandible into a protrusive position leads to the disappearance of the click because the head of the condyle is similarly guided into a protruded position, thereby gaining a more normal functional relationship to the disc. It is thought that this protective position eliminates trauma to the disc and permits the natural elasticity of the posterior part of the disc to reposition it and 'pull it' back into place.

To be effective the splint must be worn full time. During the period of splint usage, the patient should remove it only for cleaning after meals. The splint should be retained in the mouth when eating.

Some authors suggested that after wearing ARPS for 24 hours, some patients were generally not able to retrude their mandible to maximum

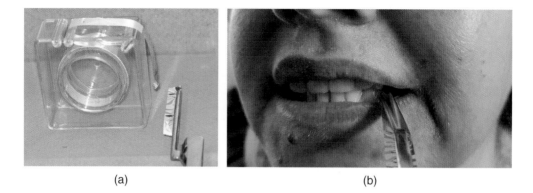

(a)   (b)

Figure 5.11 (a) Shimstock held with Millers forceps. (b) The maximum intercuspation contacts in patient's mouth being checked with shimstock. (M. Ziad Al-Ani, Robin J.M. Gray.)

intercuspation because of the possibility of contracture of lateral ptery-goid muscle, proliferation of soft tissue posterior to the condyles, remod-elling of condyles, and/or dentolalveolar changes.

It is recommended, therefore, that patients wear ARPS should be followed to review their progress at regular intervals and to determine whether they begin to lose their ability to occlude into centric occlusion. This can be observed by recording shim stock hold occlusal record before and during the treatment with ARPS (Figure 5.11).

If patient starts to lose their ability to hold shim stock, compared to the initial stock hold record, they should immediately discontinue using the splint.

After the 24/7, three-month wear, there is a controlled and gradual weaning-off period. This is done on a gradual basis by leaving the splint out during the day for an hour in the morning and an hour in the after-noon, then 2 hours, 3 hours, and so on, gradually building up these peri-ods until the appliance is not worn at all during the day. During this period, it should still be worn at night. Once successful weaning off dur-ing the day has occurred, which usually takes two to three weeks, the splint can be left out at night, leaving it out one night a week, then two nights a week and, so on, alternating the nights as far as possible. Once the splint is worn for only approximately 50% of the nights, its usage can be discontinued.

This splint has been shown to be highly successful in 85–90% of patients, producing an improvement or resolution of the clicking. Patients should be advised that they will never do themselves any harm by wearing the splint and should the click recur there is no contraindication to going back to wearing the appliance for a period of time, as long as it has remained a good fit, and subsequently slowing down the weaning-off process.

Give supportive and dietary advice. Initially, the splint will cause prob-lems with speech, but these will be overcome in a surprisingly short space of time – usually 36–48 hours. Eating is difficult initially, so give a diet sheet suggesting pasta, eggs, fish mince, soups, and so forth. Reassure your patients that they will get back to a more normal diet quite quickly. An altered softer diet is also part of the treatment, thereby reducing the load on the TMJs.

Other proposed treatments for disc displacement with reduction, such as splint therapy followed by a second phase of treatment involving orthodontic or restorative treatment to establish a new relationship between the jaws, are very rarely if ever indicated as are arthrocentesis and surgery and are out with the remit of this text.

The patient journey

History and examination 1

This is a two-way procedure. Consider all aspects and listen to your patient who will give you the diagnosis. Keep your ears and eyes open.

Special tests

Narrow your thoughts down and focus on what you really need.

Think of radiographs as being an aid to diagnosis rather than a necessity, and request them only when essential.

Diagnosis

Think of all the possibilities. This patient has a consistent not an intermittent click, which has recently started to cause discomfort. She has an internal derangement of disc replacement with reduction and secondary muscle tenderness. Rationalise that you have reached a sensible diagnosis on which to base a treatment plan that is practical and economically possible for you to undertake in your practice should you so wish.

Treatment

Consider the practical options then come to a conclusion.

One option is to do nothing if she is unconcerned but keep her under review. She might be resistant to wearing a splint and just wants reassurance. She might be worried about the consequences of leaving the condition untreated and requests active intervention. Adapt your treatment plan to the patient's needs and avoid being prescriptive and using the 'one condition – one treatment' approach.

Advice and reassurance

This is important! Explain that jaw joint clicking is very common and, in the absence of pain and restriction of movement, not a major problem. Explain the anatomical and physiological basis of the click. Explain about grinding and clenching. Talk about physiotherapy referral if there is muscle tenderness and give dietary advice.

Splint treatment 7

Always advise evidence-based treatments. You know that the ARPS has a high success rate. You must stress the importance of 24-hours-a-day wear for 12 weeks. Talk about diet and the need for excellent OH. Exclude partial coverage appliances.

Result

A well thought out treatment plan and a happy patient!

Further Reading

Clark, G.T. (1984). Treatment of jaw clicking with temporomandibular repositioning: analysis of 25 cases. *Cranio* 2: 263–270.

Clark, G.T. (1986). The TMJ repositioning appliance: a technique for construction, insertion, and adjustment. *Cranio* 4: 37–46.

Davies, S.J. and Gray, R.J.M. (1997). The pattern of splint usage in the management of two common temporomandibular disorders. Part I: the anterior repositioning splint in the treatment of disc displacement with reduction. *Br Dent J* 183: 199–203.

Davies, S.J. and Gray, R.J.M. (1997). The pattern of splint usage in the management of two common temporomandibular disorders. Part III: long-term follow-up in an assessment of splint therapy in the management of disc displacement with reduction and pain dysfunction syndrome. *Br Dent J* 183: 279–283.

de Senna, B.R., dos Santos Silva, V.K. et al. (2009). Imaging diagnosis of the temporomandibular joint: critical review of indications and new perspectives. *Oral Radiol* 25: 86–98.

Eliasson, S. and Isacsson, G. (1992). Radiographic signs of temporomandibular disorders to predict outcome of treatment. *J Craniomandib Disord* 6: 281–287.

Epstein, J.B., Caldwell, J., and Black, G. (2001). The utility of panoramic imaging of the temporomandibular joint in patients with temporomandibular disorders. *Oral Surg Oral Med Oral Pathol Oral Radiol Endod* 92: 236–239.

Gray, R.J.M., Quayle, A.A., Horner, K., and Al-Gorashi, A.J. (1991). The effects of positioning variations in transcranial radiographs of the temporomandibular joint: a laboratory study. *Br J Oral Maxillofac Surg* 29: 241–249.

Horner, K and Eaton, K.A. (2018). *Selection Criteria for Dental Radiography*, 3rd Edition. London: Faculty of General Dental Practitioners.

The Ionising Radiation (Medical Exposure) Regulations 2018. Available at: https://www.legislation.gov.uk/uksi/2018/121/introduction/made.

Lundh, H., Westesson, P., Kopp, S., and Tillström, B. (1985). Anterior repositioning splint in the treatment of temporomandibular joints with reciprocal clicking: comparison with a flat occlusal splint and an untreated control group. *Oral Surg Oral Med Oral Pathol* 60: 131–136.

Simma, I., Gleditsch, J.M., Simma, L., and Piehslinger, E. (2009). Immediate effects of microsystem acupuncture in patients with oromyofascial pain and craniomandibular disorders (CMD): a double-blind, placebo-controlled trial. *Br Dent J* 207 (12): E26.

Simmons, H.C. 3rd and Gibbs, S.J. (2009). Anterior repositioning appliance therapy for TMJ disorders: specific symptoms believed and relationship to disk status on MRI. *J Tenn Dent Assoc* 89 (4): 22–30. quiz 30–1.

Smith, P., Mosscrop, D., Davies, S. et al. (2007). The efficacy of acupuncture in the treatment of temporomandibular joint myofascial pain: a randomized controlled trial. *J Dent* 35: 259–267.

Westesson, P.L., Cohen, J.M., and Tallents, R.H. (1991). Magnetic resonance imaging of temporomandibular joint after surgical treatment of internal derangement. *Oral Surg Oral Med Oral Pathol* 71: 407–411.

Wright, E.F. and Klasser, G.D. (2019). *Manual of Temporomandibular Disorders*, 4the. Hoboken, NJ: Whiley Blackwell.

Evidence-based Dentistry

Minakuchi, H., Kuboki, T., Malsuka, Y. et al. (2002). Patients with anterior disk displacement improve with minimal treatment. *Evidence-Based Dent* 3: 69.

Santacatterina, A., Paoli, M., Peretta, R. et al. (2000). Repositioning splint more effective than bite plane in the treatment of TMJ disk dislocation with reduction. *Evidence-Based Dent* 2: 15.

Schmitter, M., Zahran, M., Duc, J.M. et al. (2006). Centric splints more effective than distraction splints in anterior disc displacement without reduction? *Evidence-Based Dent* 7: 50.

Chapter 6

I've Got a Locking Joint

History

Katie is a 16-year-old schoolgirl who comes into your surgery in a panic with her mum first thing in the morning. She says that her jaw is locked on the right side and she can't open her mouth beyond a couple of fingers' width. She has tried to force her jaw open but this was extremely painful, and she couldn't manage it.

Previously, she had had intermittent clicking for about six months.

She had mentioned this to you at her routine examination, but at that time, the click was not present and you suggested that she should report back to you if it became a problem. She wasn't aware of what had caused the click but said that it had had a gradual onset with no particular initiating event. Over the last week, she had been aware of intermittent locking on waking in the morning, but this was always momentary and freed spontaneously within a few seconds. This morning she woke with her jaw locked. It did not free up as usual and has been locked since. She commented that since her jaw was locked the click had now gone but her jaw was very painful. She is really worried as she has exams soon and she said, 'I don't need this just now'.

She is worried not only about the pain but also about how any treatment will interfere with her studies. She attended with her mother who expressed concern about how you were going to help her today, in the immediate future and what the potential for this happening again was. Apart from her temporomandibular joint (TMJ) click, there was no relevant previous medical or dental history.

Temporomandibular Disorders: A Problem-Based Approach, Second Edition. M. Ziad Al-Ani and Robin J.M. Gray.
© 2021 M. Ziad Al-Ani and Robin J.M. Gray. Published 2021 by John Wiley & Sons Ltd.
Companion Website: www.wiley.com/go/al-ani/temporomandibular-disorders-2e

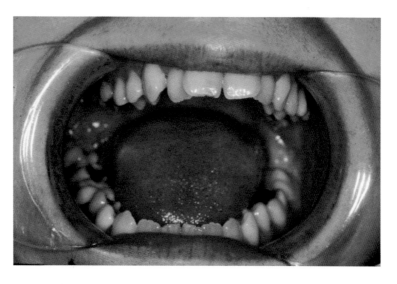

Figure 6.1 Locked right TMJ with lasting mandibular deviation. (M. Ziad Al-Ani, Robin J.M. Gray.)

Examination 1

Katie has a class I, basal bone and incisal relationship. She appeared anxious but said that when she was at rest she was not in much pain. The discomfort was present only when she tried to open her mouth beyond a certain point (Figure 6.1).

You examined the TMJs for tenderness. There was no tenderness on lateral palpation, but there was tenderness on intra-auricular palpation on the right-hand side. You palpated and listened to the jaw joints for sounds; there was no evidence of clicking. You palpated the masseter, lateral pterygoid and temporalis muscles, but there was no tenderness. Katie did comment that when she bit hard together she experienced pain in her right ear. You asked her to open her mouth and you examined her pathway of jaw movement. She could open comfortably to 17 mm, at which stage, she said her jaw 'would not go any further'. At this point, when she did try to force her mouth open further, her mandible deviated across toward the right-hand side. She said that she felt that this was because there was something 'getting in the way'. Her limitation of mouth opening was therefore not purely due to pain – there was also a physical obstruction.

Radiographs/Imaging

Katie asked you to take a radiograph because she wanted to see what was wrong. You declined to do this because you knew that a radiograph would not give you any more information and would not even confirm your clinical diagnosis.

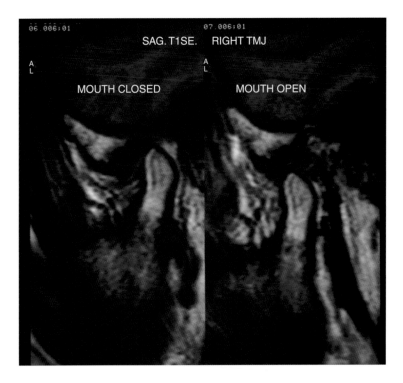

Figure 6.2 A magnetic resonance scan showing the condyle–disc relationship. (M. Ziad Al-Ani, Robin J.M. Gray.)

Further imaging such as magnetic resonance imaging (MRI) (Figure 6.2) might be suggested but only if an invasive, possibly surgical treatment plan was being contemplated, otherwise there is no indication for such a test.

MRI of the TMJ is a proven method for the assessment of hard and soft tissues and is rapidly surpassing arthrography and computed tomography (CT) as the imaging method of choice. The major advantages of MRI in comparison to arthrography and CT are that

- It is non-invasive.
- It requires no ionizing radiation for image acquisition.
- Multiplanar imaging is readily obtained and more easily interpretable.

In contrast, the disadvantages are

- High initial cost of the scanner.
- Special site planning.
- Shielding danger to patients with cerebral aneurysm clips, pacemakers, metallic prosthetic heart valves, or pregnant patients (in the first trimester).

The posterior band of the disc is characteristically located superior to the condyle and in the glenoid fossa. The second landmark for normal disc

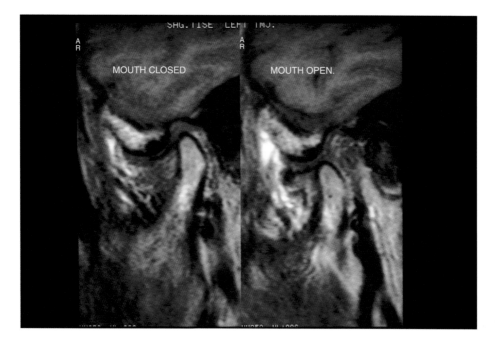

Figure 6.3 MRI can distinguish the disc from its posterior attachment. (M. Ziad Al-Ani, Robin J.M. Gray.)

position is the relationship between the anterior aspect of the condyle and the central thin zone of the disc inferiorly. These two surfaces should be close together. Separation of the anterior surface of the condyle and the central thin zone of the disc of more than a few millimetres is an indication of disc displacement. The lateral pterygoid muscles are frequently seen in the images attaching to the condyle and sometimes to the disc anteriorly. The disc has a relatively low signal, and the posterior disc attachment has a higher signal than the disc itself because of higher water content. MRI can distinguish the disc from its posterior attachment. This is a unique feature of this technique, since other techniques, such as arthrography and CT, cannot accurately differentiate the disc from its attachment (Figure 6.3).

Diagnosis

The diagnosis in Katie's case is one of an internal derangement in the TMJ of disc displacement *without* reduction. When considering this definition, think of the word 'reduction' in an anatomical way – a structure going back into place – and do not link the word reduction with reduced movement. A useful analogy is, if a shoulder joint has been dislocated, reduction of this dislocation means that the joint components are repositioned to their anatomically correct position. The correct definition of clicking is disc displacement with reduction, i.e. the disc reduces to a normal position, whereas in locking this does not happen, hence the term 'disc displacement without reduction'.

The main complaint is one of an inability to open the mouth beyond a certain degree due to a physical obstruction. Patients with this condition frequently report that trying to open their mouth causes a feeling like stretching an elastic band in the joint.

They can close their mouth freely but biting together can be painful. The reason for this is that, when a patient with an anteriorly displaced disc bites firmly in centric occlusion, as the disc is displaced forward, the highly innervated elastic posterior portion of the disc becomes interposed between the head of the condyle and the fossa. When the patient bites down, this sensitive part of the disc is 'pinched' between the bony components of the joint and is painful.

Locking must not be confused with dislocation, which is a rare occurrence and usually happens after trauma to a patient with an open mouth. In the case of dislocation, the head of the condyle moves to an abnormal degree over the articular eminence, and the resultant upward and backward muscle pull prevents its return to the glenoid fossa.

On rare occasions, there can be an anatomical predisposition to dislocation. The clinical presentation of this is a patient locked with the mouth open, usually quite wide, and deviated, usually toward one side. Locking, however, presents with opposite symptoms. It is not normally a painful condition unless the patient tries to open wide.

Treatment

How should Katie's condition be managed? She is worried that she might need 'an operation'.

The primary treatment for disc displacement without reduction is generally conservative. As always counselling is the first stage of treatment. She should be advised to consciously restrict her range of mouth movement. She should strictly adhere to a soft diet. If there is a specific area of pain then an anti-inflammatory topical gel can be applied, as can hot and cold compresses.

 Physiotherapy should be your first treatment line in a musculoskeletal disorder and can take the form of outpatient electrophysiotherapy. The ideal regimen is two to three times a week for three to four weeks, totalling 10–12 sessions in all. The normally employed physiotherapy modalities are ultrasound, acupuncture, and megapulse. The physiotherapy should be directed at relaxation of the superior pterygoid muscle on the affected side, thereby allowing the natural elasticity of the disc to reposition it. Katie should also be counselled that spontaneous remission may occur. If the clicking starts again spontaneously or as a result of treatment, this is a good sign and she should not be alarmed because it merely means that the head of the condyle is now able to move past the disc and her range of movement will have improved.

In her case, the history of the complaint is very short so treatment could include muscle relaxant therapy alongside physiotherapy. Muscle relaxant therapy should take the form of Temazepam Oral Suspension 10 mg taken at night as a maximum dose. Ideally, as little as possible should be taken to produce relaxation and lessen the symptoms while avoiding drowsiness or other side effects. It should be remembered that this drug is licensed as an anxiolytic, although it also has a pharmacologically recognised muscle relaxant effect. It appears to have an effect by relaxing contraction of the pterygoid muscles, thereby allowing the disc to reposition. Prescription of this drug, especially in an adolescent, should be undertaken either by her GP or with her general medical practitioner's knowledge and consent. She should be advised to take this 30 minutes before retiring at night and to titrate the dose herself so that she not only wakes without discomfort, but also with no unwanted side effects. She should take this drug only for five to seven days initially before you reassess her. Temazepam cannot be prescribed for patients aged under 12 years.

If temazepam oral suspension is to be prescribed privately, the clinician must apply to their primary care trust for a special form for prescription (FP10PCD) as temazepam is a controlled drug.

 If locking is of very recent onset, it is sometimes possible to manipulate the mandible to free the disc. This is done by asking the patient to bite with a wooden tongue spatula between the molar teeth on the affected side for approximately one minute. This causes the muscles on the contra-lateral side to pull the condyle up while the condyle on the affected side is 'fixed'. The patient is then asked to open the mouth gently and the operator places his/her thumbs on the molar teeth and exerts gentle downwards and posterior pressure on the affected side, while rotating the other side upwards and slightly forwards (Figure 6.4a,b).

This does work on occasion in freeing the disc, but the patient should be told that the disc is unstable. This must be followed by a period of a strict soft diet and reduction of mouth opening as far as possible.

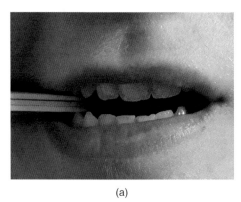
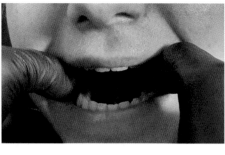

(a)   (b)

Figure 6.4 (a, b) Asking the patient to bite on a wooden tongue spatula between the molar teeth on the affected side for approximately one minute followed by manipulation may be a helpful procedure in freeing the disc. (M. Ziad Al-Ani, Robin J.M. Gray.)

If she returns to clicking, you might consider construction of an anterior repositioning splint, once the acute phase has settled. If conservative measures fail, referral to a specialist clinic should be made before any further treatment is considered.

Exercises are often prescribed and patients also feel that they should vigorously move their jaw to 'loosen it up!' This is wrong. Exercise and forced movement should be strictly avoided during the acute phase because of the risk of damaging the displaced disc even further. Once the acute symptoms have settled, corrective exercise can be prescribed to remedy abnormal mandibular movement pathways.

If the disc remains out of position and her lock shows no sign of resolving after a 12- to 16-week period, manipulation of the mandible under a general anaesthetic may become an option. It is difficult to put a timescale on when such a decision should be made because this will be an individual judgement made by the patient, her parents (if appropriate) and the clinician together.

Arthrocentesis or joint lavage is another recognised treatment modality if the lock persists. The pressure of fluid injected into the joint during this washing-out process may facilitate joint movements by releasing or breaking intracapsular adhesions. Removal of inflammatory mediators in the joint by arthrocentesis may also contribute to a reduction in the symptoms.

On rare occasions when the locking is long term, appears permanent, no spontaneous improvement has occurred, and there is no response to any conservative treatment, surgery may be an option. This should be considered only if the symptoms are totally unacceptable to the patient on a day-to-day basis, if there is imaging evidence confirming the disc displacement and all conservative measures have failed.

A recent systematic review of the management of disc displacement without reduction recommended using the simplest, least costly, and least invasive interventions for the initial management as there was insufficient evidence to support or refute the use of minimally invasive and invasive surgical interventions in these cases.

TMJ locking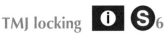

The term 'locking' refers to the common clinical presentation described in Katie's case.

This term describes a situation where the patient can open to a limited degree but no further. Movement, both opening and closing, can usually occur freely up to the point at which locking occurs. The patient then describes a distinct sense of sticking within the joint, which can be very painful in the acute phase, but otherwise is often less so, indicating that the restriction is primarily due to a physical obstruction rather than pain.

In this situation, the disc is usually displaced anteromedially to such a degree that the bilaminar zone is stretched considerably and thinned. The condyle is located behind the thick posterior band of the disc which

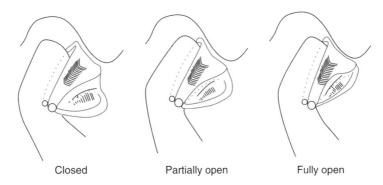

Closed   Partially open   Fully open

Figure 6.5 Anteriorly displaced non-reducing disc in relation to condyle during mouth opening. (Gray RJ, Davies SJ, Quayle AA. A clinical approach to temporomandibular disorders. 2. Examination of the articulatory system: the temporomandibular joints. Br Dent J 1994;176:473–7,© 1994, Springer Nature.)

tends to bunch up anteriorly. Locking then occurs because the position and distortion of the disc are such that the condyle is unable to gain access to the undersurface of the disc during mouth opening (Figure 6.5).

While rotation of the condyle can still occur, allowing an incisal opening of about 17–20 mm, translation is prevented. Mouth opening can improve spontaneously with the passage of time, which may be due to either reduction of the disc displacement that would be accompanied by return of the click, or gradual stretching of the attachments of the disc, in which case there would be no joint sounds. In this latter situation, a near normal range of mouth opening can be attained in time, but this is usually still accompanied by deviation towards the affected side. There can be other rare causes such as the head of the condyle locating into a perforation in the intra-articular disc; this, however, is very unusual.

How important is measuring the range of movement?

Jaw movements are the only parameters that can be objectively recorded and measured. Mouth opening is important not only as a record of the severity of the symptoms but also as an indication of the rate and degree of improvement. It has been shown that this parameter was the only valid measurement in discriminating between patients with or without a TMD.

Discriminating between a reduction in the range of vertical movement as a result of a muscular problem and one caused by of a physical obstruction is essential in making an accurate diagnosis of the TMD. The reduction in movement due to pain only is most likely to indicate a muscular problem, whereas limited mouth opening as a result of a physical obstruction is indicative of disc displacement. It has been suggested that even a moderate reduction in mouth opening may indicate a TMD, so it is recommended that this variable should be routinely recorded. The normal range of movement has been suggested as being 35 mm for females and 42 mm for males and 8 mm in either direction for lateral excursion.

Conclusion

In Katie's case, as the disc displacement was acute, and she had presented very rapidly for the treatment, she responded well to outpatient physiotherapy which consisted of ultrasound three times a week for three weeks and temazepam 10 mg at night for seven days. Her click returned and her jaw freed. You discussed with her the option of further treatment and she elected to have an anterior repositioning splint but wanted to wait until her exams were over.

Further Reading

Frost, D.E., Kendell, B.D., and Part, I.I. (1999). The use of arthrocentesis for treatment of temporomandibular joint disorders. *J Oral Maxillofac Surg* 57.

Gray, R.J.M., Quayle, A.A., Hall, C.A., and Schofield, M.A. (1994). Physiotherapy in the treatment of temporomandibular joint disorders: a comparative study of four treatment methods. *Br Dent J* 176: 257–261.

Kai, S., Kai, H., Tabata, O. et al. (1998). Long-term outcomes of nonsurgical treatment in nonreducing anteriorly displaced disk of the temporomandibular joint. *Oral Surg Oral Med Oral Pathol Oral Radiol Endod* 85: 258–267.

Nicolakis, P., Erdogmus, B., Kopf, A. et al. (2001). Effectiveness of exercise therapy in patients with internal derangement of the temporomandibular joint. *J Oral Rehabil* 28: 1158–1164.

Shi, Z., Guo, C., and Awad, M. (2003). Hyaluronate for temporomandibular joint disorders. *Cochrane Database Systemat Rev* 1: CD002970.

Evidence-based Dentistry

Al-Baghdadi, M., Durham, J., Araujo-Soares, V. et al. (2014). TMJ disc displacement without reduction management: a systematic review. *J Dent Res* 93 (7 Suppl): 37S–51S.

Schiffman, E.L., Look, J.O., Hodges, J.S. et al. (2007). Non-surgical care should be the primary treatment for TMJ closed lock. *Evidence-Based Dent* 8: 112.

Chapter 7

I've Got a Grating Joint

Mrs Smith is a patient whom you have known for several years. She has attended for routine examinations; she wears partial upper and lower acrylic dentures that are old and worn and have poor occlusion. She is missing most of her posterior teeth in both arches. Her dentures are several years old, and she is now lacking posterior support. She is 67 years of age and, although you have encouraged her in the past to get new dentures, she wishes to continue with the ones that she has because she feels that she is too old to adapt to something new.

She has attended for her six-monthly examination and mentions to you in passing that she has discomfort in her left ear. She said that she has had a crunching or grating noise in her ear when she moves her jaw for four or five years, but she has recently become aware of discomfort. She feels that her mouth opening is restricted; she has no pain on waking, but feels that her discomfort comes on with function and gets worse as the day goes on. She says that her jaw feels 'heavy'. She does not get headaches and says that the pain is located to the area immediately in front of her ear and 'is in my ear'. She has osteoarthrosis and is awaiting admission to hospital for a hip replacement. She has also recently been diagnosed with breast cancer and has had a general anaesthetic for a lumpectomy. The pathology has been reported as being a benign lump. She had a mastectomy 12 years ago and underwent a course of radiotherapy and chemotherapy. She is taking tamoxifen and an antidepressant. She is a retired teacher.

Examination

She has a class II, division I, basal bone and incisal relationship. She has an overjet of 6 mm, and she is now aware of having to posture her jaw

Temporomandibular Disorders: A Problem-Based Approach, Second Edition. M. Ziad Al-Ani and Robin J.M. Gray.
© 2021 M. Ziad Al-Ani and Robin J.M. Gray. Published 2021 by John Wiley & Sons Ltd.
Companion Website: www.wiley.com/go/al-ani/temporomandibular-disorders-2e

forwards to be able to chew but this is uncomfortable. She feels that she has a restricted range of movement, only being able to open comfortably to two finger widths. You measured this as 25 mm. The left temporomandibular joint (TMJ) is tender on lateral and intra-auricular palpation. You examined the temporalis and masseter muscles digitally and the lateral pterygoid muscles against resistance. She has no obvious masticatory muscle tenderness. Even without the use of a stethoscope you were able to hear a crepitation or grating noise from her left TMJ when she opened her mouth widely. Mrs Smith reported that she felt that her bite had changed somewhat but you are unable to detect any significant occlusal abnormalities because of the poor occlusion of her dentures. This was also because she was very 'hand shy', as she did not want you to palpate her TMJ, and because she could not comfortably move her mandible from side to side. You found it very difficult to establish her centric jaw relationship.

She was very anxious about her symptoms because of her previous history of breast cancer as she felt that she might have a tumour. She insisted on you referring her for a radiograph.

 Although you would not normally have required a radiograph, you agreed to do so in this instance because there was good reason to allay her very obvious anxiety and, in the circumstances, you felt that this test was justifiable.

Radiographic examination

You requested a DPT. This showed a normal outline of the mandibular condyle on the right side but showed loss of the condylar outline of the mandibular condyle on the left side and sclerosis of the articular fossa (Figure 7.1).

Diagnosis

Your diagnosis was osteoarthrosis in the TMJ on the left side.

Treatment

It is suggested the natural history and progress of osteoarthrosis from the first clinical sign to the final subsidence of pain and stiffness, if untreated, can vary from one year to three years, but on occasion, the condition may take longer to stabilise and symptoms to improve. Simple symptomatic treatment gives encouragement and makes the disease more tolerable for the patient. Most patients with osteoarthrosis of the TMJ do not appear to have significant problems; it is mainly acute exacerbations and reduced range of movement that necessitate active intervention. In Mrs Smith's case, she was aware of the crepitation which had been present for years.

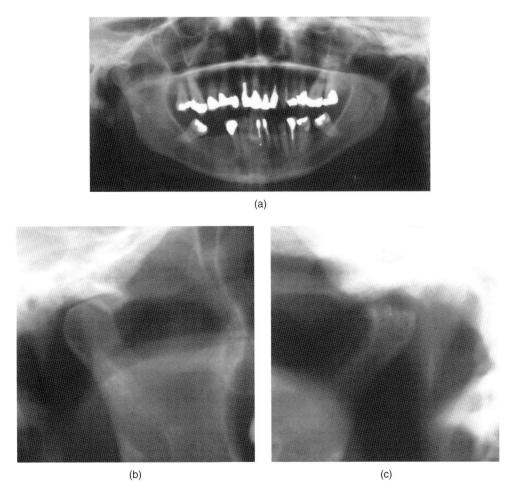

(a)

(b)   (c)

Figure 7.1 (a) Dental panoramic tomogram; (b) close-up of normal joint right; (c) close-up of degenerative joint disease left. (M. Ziad Al-Ani, Robin J.M. Gray.)

This did not concern her, and you and she had talked about it before. What was new, however, was the discomfort and difficulty with chewing. These were her immediate concerns.

The latest Cochrane systematic review on the interventions for managing temporomandibular joint osteoarthrosis found a lack of data from randomised controlled trials which makes decision-making about the management of osteoarthrosis of the TMJ 'strongly dependent on consumers' preferences and clinical expertise

Explanation and reassurance

Patients are encouraged by the fact that this disease often improves spontaneously as the TMJ retains the capacity to repair and remodel throughout life. It should be explained that symptoms may worsen before they

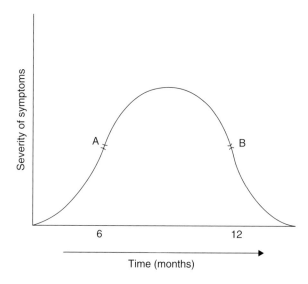

Figure 7.2 Diagrammatic presentation of the progress of osteoarthrosis symptoms. (Ogus MD, Toller P. Common Disorders of the Temporomandibular Joint. Bristol: John Wright & Sons Ltd, 1981 © 1981, John Wright & Sons Ltd.)

improve. A useful way of illustrating this is to draw a graph or curve which will assist in explaining the prognosis of the condition (Figure 7.2).

It is conceded that at the time of consultation, it may be difficult to assess the patient's precise position on the curve. Therefore, if the current stage is at point A, a period of deterioration will precede improvement. If on the other hand it is at point B, the condition is on its way to resolving. At the initial visit there is little way of predicting the immediate future pathway of the symptoms unless the patient volunteers they are generally improving or alternatively, deteriorating.

Physiotherapy

Voluntary immobilisation such as reduction of mouth opening, i.e. stifling a yawn, heat and gentle massage are useful modalities included in a physiotherapy regimen. Joint rest is a functional tenet of arthritic therapy and with the TMJ can be achieved by varying degrees of controlled joint immobilisation, usually involving a soft diet and voluntary avoidance of excessive mandibular movement. Electrophysiotherapy can include ultrasound, Megapulse, acupuncture, or soft laser treatment. Soft laser has a recognised effect on fibroblast production and can stimulate healing. A non-steroidal anti-inflammatory gel rubbed into the skin over the affected sites can also be helpful. Several jaw exercises have been suggested. These should be avoided during the acute phase. Mrs Smith was happy to have a course of outpatient physiotherapy, so you arranged this. You stressed that the course must be intensive, i.e. two to three sessions a week for three to four weeks totalling 10–12 sessions in all. Attending once a week or irregularly would have little lasting benefit.

Medication

Pain relief forms a major part of treatment and, assuming that there are no contraindications, non-steroidal anti-inflammatory drugs are useful. It should be pointed out, however, that there is no evidence to suggest that the natural history of osteoarthrosis is significantly affected by these drugs; they are used for control of pain and inflammation.

Mrs Smith was anxious to avoid taking medication if it could be avoided – 'I am not a pill person!'

Reduction of contributory predisposing factors

Some authors refer to a possible correlation between the number of opposing posterior occlusal units and the occurrence of osteoarthrosis symptoms and suggest that dental treatment such as restoration of missing functional units may help. There is, however, a lack of conclusive evidence to support this claim. You had already discussed new dentures, but this suggestion was declined. Your alternative would have been to temporarily build up the occlusion of the existing dentures with light-cured or cold-cure acrylic to re-establish posterior contact, because this could have had a beneficial effect. Symptomatic treatment was, however, her preferred option.

Final treatment plan

Mrs Smith declined medication and adjustment to her dentures. She had nine sessions of Megapulse and her discomfort resolved. The crepitus remained unchanged, but this was of no concern to her.

What is crepitation? 4

Crepitation is usually reported by the patient as a grating, grinding, or crunching noise that may be audible during all jaw movements. Crepitus is usually sensed by the patient and can often be felt by the examining finger. It is audible on auscultation and varies from fine crepitation to a course staccato crunch, which on occasion can be heard without the need for a stethoscope.

Is osteoarthrosis always associated with pain and crepitus? 4

In the early stages of osteoarthrosis, patients are often free from symptoms, but may have signs such as a reduced range of movement and mild (to the patient) inexplicable joint sounds – squeaking, grinding, crunching, or grating. Some joints with structural changes characteristic of osteoarthrosis are clinically asymptomatic.

As osteoarthrosis of a TMJ progresses the following signs and symptoms may be observed:

- Aching that is usually initially localised to the area of the joint but can subsequently radiate over the affected side of the face due to secondary muscle symptoms.
- Pain on movement of the jaw, not only on biting or attempted wide opening, but that can be present at any part of the range of movement. The pain is sometimes of a persistent aching character at rest, but is exacerbated by jaw movement.
- Tenderness over the TMJ particularly with the mouth open and when palpation is directed towards the back of the condyle.
- A reduced range of jaw movement is a common feature of osteoarthrosis, not necessarily on waking in the morning. This symptom, in addition to pain, tends to become worse with function. The reason for this is because the structure of the joint is damaged, and this joint therefore has a reduced capacity even for normal load. In this instance, even normal function will cause symptoms.

The normal clinical picture is for osteoarthrosis of the TMJ to affect one side only. It has been suggested that joint stiffness and limitation of jaw movement are mainly a result of secondary inflammation of the capsular tissues. On very rare occasions, when there has been loss of condylar height, occlusal changes may result because of shortening of the ascending ramus. A tilting of the occlusal plane occasionally associated with deviation towards the affected side can occur. Even less frequently an anterior open bite may result; this, however, is highly unusual and usually associated with rheumatoid arthritis.

Pyrophosphate can be found in high concentrations in synovial fluid in joints with osteoarthrosis. Calcium crystals can be formed from the combination of pyrophosphate and calcium, which may subsequently provoke an acute inflammatory response with consequent pain and impairment of the normal free-sliding, low-friction movement of the jaw.

Radiographic changes

The TMJ is a difficult joint to examine using simple radiographic techniques. Its position within the dense skull base makes straightforward imaging difficult. The normal way to view the TMJ is laterally, but this leads to superimposition from the contralateral joint and partial obscuring by the petrous temporal bone of the skull base. Simple radiographic techniques, therefore use oblique beams in an attempt to find an unobstructed pathway for the X-ray beam to achieve a useful result.

In early disease, radiological features may be undetected. Studies have reported variable frequencies of radiological signs; however, many of these abnormalities disappear with time, probably reflecting remodelling associated with growth and repair. There tend to be two common radiological presentations: degenerative, when erosion and loss of the condylar outline are apparent, or, in contrast, when there is marked proliferative change with osteophyte formation and sclerosis. On tomography, the earliest detectable changes in osteoarthrosis are surface erosions associated with damage to the subarticular cortical bone. Osteophytes are occasionally seen in the later stages and usually present at the anterior aspect of the condyle, although occasionally on the lateral margin. Lipping has, however, been observed without any other evidence of pathological changes, so the presence of a bony spur evident on a radiograph may be irrelevant if no other signs or symptoms are present. Anterior lipping of the mandibular condyle may represent a progressive remodelling process in response to changing functional demands often associated with increasing age, and may not necessarily be indicative of osteoarthrosis. It is accepted that the mandibular condyle even with an osteophyte can function efficiently, free from symptoms and with no alteration to the occlusion.

As the disease progresses radiographically, loss of the condylar cortical outline and erosion become more pronounced. With progress of the disease into the reparative phase the anterior aspect of the mandibular condyle becomes flattened and the outline more pyramidal than rounded.

It should be remembered that radiographic changes appear to develop some months after the clinical symptoms. A comparison of clinical features, radiographic findings, and subsequent histology suggests that if TMJ symptoms are severe the pathological damage to the articular surface of the condyle at a cellular level is more advanced than radiographs might indicate.

Treatment of pathological sequelae

A minority of patients with an osteoarthritic TMJ end up with prolonged discomfort and intractable pain as a result of gross pathological tissue changes. This situation is, however, rare.

Invasive treatment

Arthrocentesis One possible treatment is arthrocentesis. This involves introduction of a cannula into the joint space; it is associated with joint irrigation, with two needles within the joint space to allow continual flow of fluid in and out. Medications, such as local anaesthetics, steroids and synthetic synovial fluids, may be added during arthrocentesis. The lavage is thought to eliminate much of the secondary inflammatory mediators that produce pain.

To date, there have been many clinical studies reporting the results of TMD patients treated with arthrocentesis, and they are uniformly supportive. Arthrocentesis may be an option for the clinician to consider between failed conservative treatment and invasive surgery. In the past decade, arthrocentesis has been used with increasing frequency to treat TMJ internal derangement that failed to improve following a reasonable course of nonsurgical therapy. The clinical effectiveness of the procedure, however, has not been summarized in the form of a systematic review. Evidence demonstrates that, following arthrocenthesis, recording inflammatory medications responsible for causing pain could be eliminated. There is, however, no evidence to support the theory of this procedure being of value in disc repositioning.

Intra-articular injection of a steroid In patients with, for example, severe degenerative joint disease and severe pain, who do not respond to conservative treatment, intra-articular injection of a steroid may be used.

Injection of such drugs utilizes their powerful anti-inflammatory effect to reduce localized clinical symptoms. Several authors reported that, when symptoms are severe, then there is relief of pain and establishment of improved movement and early restoration of function following intra-articular steroid injection, without causing radiographic signs of further joint destruction. Your patient should be counselled, however, that using an 'injured joint' with symptoms artificially suppressed could cause further damage if supportive advice is not given, such as rest and strict adherence to a soft diet.

The drugs most commonly used are Triamcinolone and Depomedrone. Intra-articular steroid injections can be repeated, but it has been suggested that further erosion can occur with repeated injection.

Hyaluronate An alternative agent, with few side-effects, is sodium hyaluronate. This drug, which is injected into the joint, has also been shown to give a significant short and long-term reduction of subjective symptoms and clinical signs in patients with persistent TMJ problems that have not responded to conservative treatment. It is suggested that sodium hyaluronate can provide lubrication for the articulating surfaces and is largely responsible for synovial fluid viscosity. The latest published systematic review which assessed the effectiveness of intra-articular injection of hyaluronate, both alone and in combination with other TMD remedies, found that hyaluronate had the same short- and long-term effects on the improvement of symptoms, clinical signs or overall condition of the disorder when compared to glucocorticoids. Moreover, it has been reported that hyaluronate had a potential of improving the arthroscopic evaluation scores. The authors conclusion, however, was that there is insufficient, consistent evidence to either support or refute the use of hyaluronate for treating patients with TMD and further high-quality randomised controlled trials (RCTs) of hyaluronate need to be conducted before firm conclusions with regard to its effectiveness can be drawn.

In general, the available literature seems to be inconclusive as to the effectiveness of hyaluronate acid injections with respect to other therapeutic modalities in treating TMJ disorders.

Surgery may be a treatment option when symptoms persist and are totally unacceptable to the patient on a day-to-day basis. The surgical procedures that have been most frequently employed are an intracapsular condylectomy and a condylar shave, in which the diseased portion of bone is removed. It is thought that a new fibrous surface forms, thereby allowing the joint to function.

Arthroscopy is a less invasive approach than open joint surgery. With this technique a variety of 'surgical' procedures can be accomplished. This technique involves placing an arthroscope into the superior joint space, rendering the intracapsular structures visible on a monitor. Bone spurs can be removed with shavers and the joint space can be increased by inflation of balloon stents. This procedure has been shown to be successful in reducing symptoms and improving the range of jaw movement. Therapeutic agents can also be placed using this technique.

Further Reading

Dashnyam, K., Lee, J.H., Mandakhbayar, N. et al. (2018). Intra-articular biomaterials-assisted delivery to treat temporomandibular joint disorders. *J Tissue Eng* 9: 1–12.

de Leeuw, R., Boering, G., Stegenga, B., and de Bont, L.G. (1994). Clinical signs of TMJ osteoarthrosis and internal derangement 30 years after nonsurgical treatment. *J Orofac Pain* 8: 18–24.

González-García, R., Moreno-Sánchez, M., Moreno-García, C. et al. (2018). Arthroscopy of the inferior compartment of the temporomandibular joint: a new perspective. *J Maxillofac Oral Surg* 17: 228–232.

Gurung, T., Singh, R.K., Mohammad, S. et al. (2017). Efficacy of arthrocentesis versus arthrocentesis with sodium hyaluronic acid in temporomandibular joint osteoarthritis: a comparison. *Natl. J. Maxillofac. Surg.* 8: 41–49.

Kopp, S. (1987). Clinical findings in temporomandibular joint osteoarthrosis. *Scand J Dent Res* 85: 434–443.

Mejersjo, C. (1987). Therapeutic and prognostic considerations in TMJ osteoarthrosis: a literature review and a long-term study in 11 subjects. *Cranio* 5: 69–78.

Manfredini, D., Favero, L., Gregorini, G. et al. (2013). Natural course of temporomandibular disorders with low pain-related impairment: a 2-to-3-year follow-up study. *J Oral Rehabil.* 40: 436–442.

Ogus, M.D. and Toller, P. (1981). *Common Disorders of the Temporomandibular Joint*. John Wright & Sons Ltd: Bristol.

Soni, A. (2019). Arthrocentesis of temporomandibular joint-Bridging the gap between non-surgical and surgical treatment. *Ann Maxillofac Surg* 9 (1): 158–167.

Surya Sudhakar, G.V., Laxmi, M.S., Rahman, T., and Anand, D.S. (2018). Long-term management of temporomandibular joint degenerative changes and osteoarthritis: An attempt. *Clin Cancer Investig J* 7: 90–96.

Yoshimura, Y., Yoshida, Y., Oka, M. et al. (1982). Long-term evaluation of non-surgical treatment of osteoarthrosis of temporomandibular joint. *Int J Oral Surg* 11: 7–13.

Evidence-based Dentistry

Alpaslan, G.H. and Alpaslan, G. (2002). Arthrocentesis with sodium hyaluronate is more effective than arthrocentesis alone in temporomandibular joint treatment. *Evidence-Based Dent* 3: 70–71.

de Souza, R.F., Lovato da Silva, C.H., Nasser, M. et al. (2012). Interventions for managing temporomandibular joint osteoarthritis. *Cochrane Database Syst. Rev.* 4: CD007261.

Guo, C., Shi, Z., and Revington, P. (2009). Temporomandibular joint arthrocentesis and lavage. *Evidence-Based Dent* 10: 110.

Juniper, R. (2002). Arthrocentesis with sodium hyaluronate is more effective than arthrocentesis alone in temporomandibular joint treatment. *Evid Based Dent* 3: 70–71.

Reston, J.T. and Turkelson, C.M. (2005). Temporomandibular articular disorders can be alleviated with surgery. *Evidence-Based Dent* 6: 48–50.

Shi, Z., Guo, C., and Awad, M. (2013). Hyaluronate for temporomandibular joint disorders. *Cochrane Database Syst Rev.* 1: CD002970.

Vos, L.M., Huddleston Slater, J.J., and Stegenga, B. (2013). Lavage therapy versus nonsurgical therapy for the treatment of arthralgia of the temporomandibular joint: a systematic review of randomized controlled trials. *J Orofac Pain* 27: 171–179.

Chapter 8

You've Changed My Bite

History

Mrs Smith is a 40-year-old teacher and is a new patient to your practice. You already treat her husband and her two children. She attends complaining of pain over the right side of her face in front of her ear, headache, and a feeling of restricted jaw movement.

Mrs Smith was a regular attender at another practice close to you. She had no problems until two months ago when she started to experience facial pain after she had a bridge fitted to replace a missing upper right first and second premolar teeth. She had this bridge placed for aesthetic reasons only. She had had the teeth taken out two years ago after an abscess and a failed root canal treatment and her husband had suggested that she should have the gap filled to improve her smile.

Mrs Smith is very dentally aware and readily agreed to have the treatment done. The teeth on either side of the gap had large amalgams and she was conscious of the appearance of these in any case so she felt that this would be a good idea, not only to fill the gap but also to eliminate the appearance of unsightly restorations. The teeth on either side of the gap had been prepared uneventfully and temporary crowns had been placed but at various times both had fallen off. She phoned the practice but was told that, as the teeth were only mildly sensitive and the dentist was really busy, she should just wait until the permanent bridge was ready in a couple of weeks. At this stage, she was not aware of any change in her bite.

She returned for provision of the permanent bridge and this again proceeded uneventfully. She had this done under a local anaesthetic. Following the provision of the bridge, she felt that her 'bite felt different' and she returned to the dentist three days later (Figures 8.1 and 8.2).

By this stage, she had developed right sided facial pain.

Temporomandibular Disorders: A Problem-Based Approach, Second Edition. M. Ziad Al-Ani and Robin J.M. Gray.
© 2021 M. Ziad Al-Ani and Robin J.M. Gray. Published 2021 by John Wiley & Sons Ltd.
Companion Website: www.wiley.com/go/al-ani/temporomandibular-disorders-2e

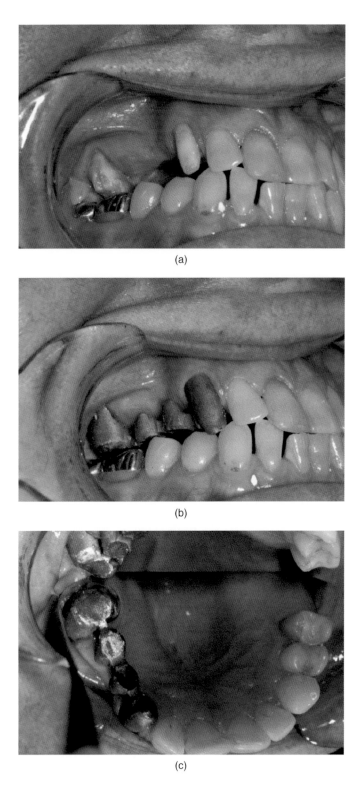

Figure 8.1 (a) Prepared bridge abutments and (b, c) heavily adjusted framework in place. (M. Ziad Al-Ani, Robin J.M. Gray.)

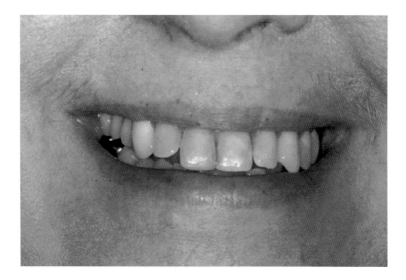

Figure 8.2 Fitted bridge: note the gap between upper and lower right lateral incisors compared with Figure 8.1a,b. (M. Ziad Al-Ani, Robin J.M. Gray.)

She said that the bridge was very sensitive to bite on and the teeth were reacting to hot and cold stimulus. However, her main complaint was that her bite felt altered. She was happy with the aesthetics of the completed restoration and to avoid any alteration to this the dentist suggested that it would be easier to adjust the bite by removing some tissue from her lower teeth opposing the bridge. The dentist did this but within a couple of days Mrs Smith was aware of the fact that her lower teeth had also become sensitive and the symptoms from the upper bridge remained unaltered. She said it was difficult to differentiate between the sensitivity she was experiencing from the bridge and from the lower teeth, but she was sure that the hypersensitivity was not restricted to the upper arch.

Mrs Smith had returned to her dentist on two subsequent occasions, and on one of these further occlusal adjustments were made, again to the lower teeth.

As the symptoms were worsening rather than improving, Mrs Smith asked her husband to book an appointment with you for a second opinion. She has decided to leave her previous practice and come to you. She commented that she felt aggrieved and she was contemplating litigation and asked for your support. She had had the bridge fitted privately and she said it 'cost an arm and a leg'. On questioning her about her medical history she said that she had been suffering from depression and was worried about 'my appearance now I have hit 40!'. She is now on an antidepressant (citalopram). She was a regular dental patient and had seen her previous dentist every six months.

Examination 1

It was apparent from intraoral examination that Mrs Smith was very dentally aware. Her oral hygiene was of a very high standard, there were no plaque or calculus deposits and her BPE was one in each sextant. All the soft tissues appeared healthy.

On examination of her articulatory system, the right TMJ was tender on lateral and especially on intra-auricular palpation. Although she felt that her mouth opening was restricted, she had a normal range of movement. Being able to open to 35 mm in the vertical dimension. This was, however, painful for her to do. There were no joint sounds.

On examination of the mandibular muscles, the right temporalis and masseter muscles were tender on palpation in the origin of both muscles, i.e. in the anterior temple and along the anterior two-thirds of the zygomatic arch. The right lateral pterygoid muscle was tender against resistance in the vertical dimension.

On examination of the occlusion, centric jaw relation and centric occlusion did not coincide, the premature contact being between the lower right first premolar and the upper right first premolar bridge pontic. The premature contact was on the mesial marginal slope of the palatal cusp of this tooth. The slide from centric relation to centric occlusion was vertical and to the left.

When examining the lateral movements of the mandible, the bridge provided interference on the non-working side on left lateral excursion. This was again against the mesial slope of the palatal cusp of the upper right first premolar pontic.

Special tests

In view of the fact Mrs Smith was a new patient to your practice, you took bite-wing radiographs and a periapical radiograph of the upper right bridge retainers. There was no adverse pathology evident.

As she had already stated to you that she was contemplating litigation, you took upper and lower impressions of her teeth and a facebow record and a centric relation occlusal record to establish her baseline occlusion. You took careful records of her teeth in the lower right quadrant opposing the bridge, as she claimed that these teeth had been adjusted. You felt that there was evidence of removal of tooth surface by a bur and took intraoral photographs of these teeth in case they should be needed later.

Treatment

In view of the potential medicolegal implications, you discussed the treatment at length with Mrs Smith to obtain her informed consent. The options that you discussed were adjusting the lower teeth, which you said you were not prepared to do, and adjusting the upper bridge, which you were happy doing but you did advise Mrs Smith that this could compromise the aesthetics. As a result of the interference on the palatal cusp, you felt that removal of the porcelain would probably expose the underlying bridge alloy metal. She was not happy with this. The third option that you discussed was removal of the bridge with replacement by an acrylic long-term provisional bridge so that this could be adjusted comfortably without change to the aesthetics, enabling Mrs Smith to regain her original comfort with her bite.

Mrs Smith said that she had felt 'a bit down recently' and wanted the fastest cure for her symptoms while not wanting to undertake treatment that would compromise her situation further. In view of her concerns about the aesthetics, you decided that removal of the bridge and replacement by provision of a temporary bridge would be the best solution. This would mean that she could enjoy the aesthetic benefits of the missing functional unit being restored and you would have time to adjust the occlusion until she was comfortable.

Mrs Smith was very happy with this because she felt that, since this problem had arisen, she had started to grind her teeth, and this was what was causing her facial pain and headache. You did explain that removal of the offending restoration could not be guaranteed to resolve her symptoms but you felt that it would be a step in the right direction. You took a rubber base impression and fabricated a chair-side temporary bridge; you did this under local anaesthetic and made an appointment the following day for Mrs Smith to return once the effects of the anaesthetic had worn off, so adjustments to the occlusion could be made to her satisfaction. At the same time, you took impressions and a jaw registration for your technician to construct a long-term provisional bridge that could be repeatedly adjusted until Mrs Smith was satisfied.

This was fitted a week later, and you managed to achieve an occlusion that Mrs Smith felt was 'as good as it was before!'

You had arranged to see her for review in a week's time, but she phoned the practice two days later to say that her symptoms had improved dramatically and that she was satisfied. You did, however, insist on seeing her at the appointed time and made further minor adjustments to the occlusion. You agreed to leave any permanent restoration for at least three months to ensure that the symptomatic improvement would be long lasting.

You saw her four months later; all her symptoms of facial pain and headache had disappeared, and she was happy with the treatment that you had provided. You removed the temporary bridge and took impressions of the upper and lower arches to forward to your technician with a careful occlusal record. The permanent bridge was fitted and no occlusal adjustments were necessary. The thermal sensitivity in the lower teeth, which had been adjusted by her previous dentist, had resolved with topical treatment and the outcome was deemed to be successful.

Discussion

A bridge made without careful consideration of the patient's occlusion is potentially hazardous. When a tooth in an arch is prepared for an indirect restoration, it is necessary to ensure that an accurate occlusal record is transmitted to your technician. A functionally stable posterior occlusion exists when enough teeth are in simultaneous even contact and occlusal forces are directed axially, thereby stabilising the position not only of the teeth but also of the TMJs. Appropriate occlusal stability distributes occlusal forces over a wide area, preventing damage to the individual components of the masticatory system. The way to achieve this is to adopt a conformative approach, which is defined as the provision of restorations 'in harmony with the existing jaw relationships'. In practice, this means that the occlusion of the new restoration is provided in such a way that the occlusal contacts of other teeth remain unaltered. The reason why this approach is favoured is not because it is the easiest, but because it is the safest. It is less likely to introduce potentially harmful consequences for the tooth, periodontium, muscles, TMJ, and patient and dentist.

Ignoring the conformative approach may result in a less-than-ideal occlusion that is not harmonious with the existing occlusion, and the patient may not tolerate this. The occlusion of the bridge that had been provided for Mrs Smith was obviously not the same as she had had pre-treatment. There was now a space between the incisal edges of the upper and lower right lateral incisors and she developed a temporo-mandibular disorder (TMD) almost immediately after this bridge was fitted.

What is notable in a patient such as Mrs Smith is that, when the occlusion was restored to the original, the symptoms disappeared rapidly. This depends on the timescale for placement of the iatrogenically introduced occlusal interference. The sooner that it is removed the quicker the symptoms will disappear.

How can this conformative approach be adopted practically?

The patient's occlusion should be recorded before any treatment is started. The construction of an indirect restoration requires the transfer of anatomical information from the clinician to the dental laboratory technician. This requires accurate models of the patient's teeth and an occlusal record, a centric jaw relation and a facebow record. Bite registration paste is better than a wax occlusal record (Figures 8.3 and 8.4).

Recently, digital technology can be utilised for the process of obtaining interocclusal recording and with the introduction of new intraoral scanner systems, virtual bite registrations can be accurately obtained (Figure 8.5).

Ideally, before tooth preparation is undertaken, occlusal contacts should be checked with articulating paper and Shimstock (Figure 8.6a–c),

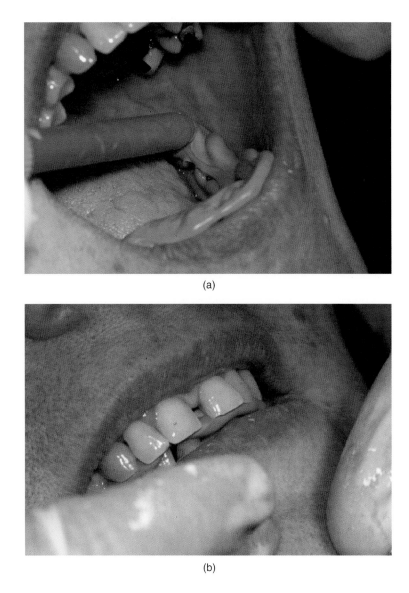

(a)

(b)

Figure 8.3 The use of a suitable material (bite registration baste) in registering a jaw relationship. (M. Ziad Al-Ani, Robin J.M. Gray.)

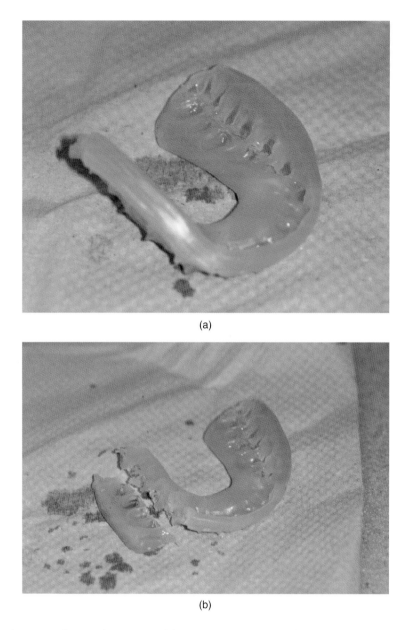

(a)

(b)

Figure 8.4 The use of a wax squashbite in registering a jaw relationship is not recommended because it readily distorts under pressure and has insufficient strength to maintain accuracy. (M. Ziad Al-Ani, Robin J.M. Gray.)

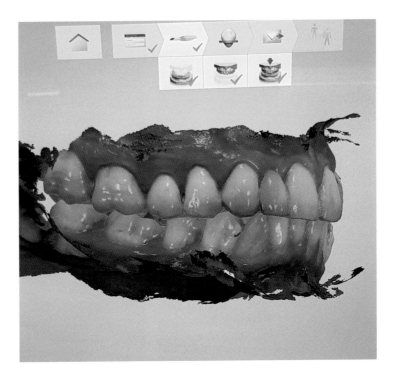

Figure 8.5 Virtual bite registrations can be accurately obtained using intraoral scanner systems. (M. Ziad Al-Ani, Robin J.M. Gray.)

not only on the teeth to be prepared but also on the adjacent teeth. A record should be made of the occlusal contacts. Unless the models exhibit exactly the same occlusal contacts as the patient's teeth, the likelihood is that the dentist will find that 'the bite is wrong' on the restoration at the fit stage. This is a not unfamiliar scenario and care at this stage will minimise, although not eliminate, the chance of error. To prevent the restoration being made on models with an inaccurate occlusion, it is important to adopt a means of checking the patient's occlusion as well as the occlusion of the models before starting the laboratory process.

An occlusal examination should record whether or not centric jaw relation/retruded contact position (CR/RCP) (Figure 8.7a,b) and centric occlusion/intercuspal position (CO/ICP), the habitual bite, are coincident. If not, where is the premature contact and is there a slide from CR to the habitual bite CO? If there is a slide, is it a large or small slide, is it in the same sagittal plane, or is it off to one side or the other? Is there anterior guidance on the canine teeth, which is the ideal, and are there any working or non-working side interferences up to and beyond the canine crossover position? These features should be recorded to enable the dentist to adhere to a conformative approach when performing restorative treatment and to have a baseline for later comparison.

It is important for the dentist to record whether there is freedom in centric occlusion. This is especially important when restoring anterior teeth

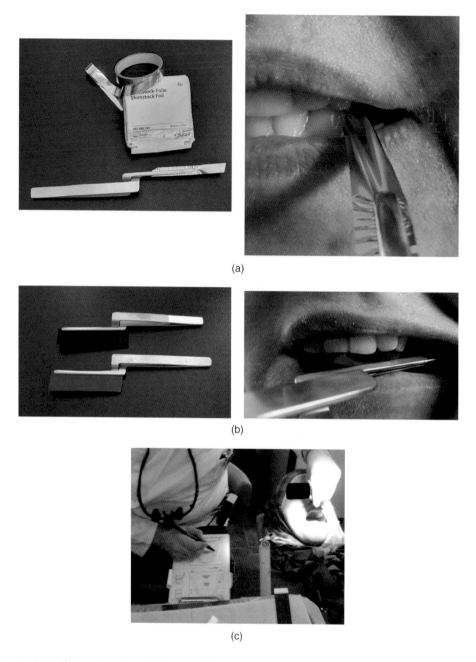

(a)

(b)

(c)

Figure 8.6 (a) Shimstock is 8 μm-thick metal foil used as a feeler gauge between occluding teeth. (b) Articulating papers held with Miller's forceps to mark occlusal contacts. (c) Recording patient's static and dynamic occlusal contacts by the dentist at the chairside. (M. Ziad Al-Ani, Robin J.M. Gray.)

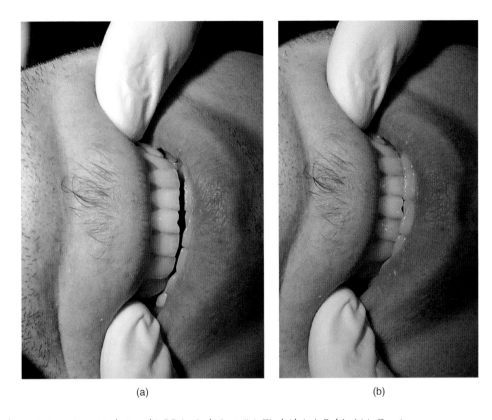

(a)   (b)

Figure 8.7 (a) CR incisal view (b) CO incisal view. (M. Ziad Al-Ani, Robin J.M. Gray.)

with, for instance, crowns, as any retrusion of the mandible by placing restorations that are thicker than the teeth were originally could cause immediate TMD symptoms or trauma to the restored teeth due to the mandible being forced distally.

Conclusion

Do you think that it was correct to leave Mrs Smith without temporary crowns even for a short period of time even though the teeth were only slightly sensitive? No!

 Do you think that the dentist adopted the correct approach by adjusting the teeth opposing the bridge to improve the occlusion and hopefully reduce the patient's discomfort? No!

This is obviously wrong and is medicolegally indefensible. It was apparent that a change in the patient's occlusion was caused by loss of the temporary crowns and/or placement of the permanent bridge to an incorrect occlusion, and this was directly responsible for the onset of the TMD symptoms. This was further reinforced by the fact that, when the occlusion was corrected by placement and subsequent adjustment of the temporary bridge, the symptoms resolved rapidly.

Mrs Smith had the bridge placed for aesthetic reasons. The occlusion was incorrect which caused a TMD. She did not want the bridge to be adjusted because the underlying alloy would have been exposed, and this would have been aesthetically unacceptable. The lower teeth should not have been adjusted under any circumstances.

A provisional bridge was made and her symptoms resolved. A final permanent restoration was constructed and Mrs Smith remained symptom free.

 Do you think that the change of occlusion of Mrs Smith has caused her a TMD?

The relationship between temporomandibular disorders and occlusion remains controversial. Some authors believe that occlusion is the primary factor in the onset of TMD symptoms, whereas others feel that occlusion has no role at all. The majority of reasoning behind causation is based upon anecdotal rather than scientific evidence and the existing evidence support the absence of a disease-specific association.

To date, most occlusal studies have assessed the static relationship of the teeth and considered the significance or non-significance of occlusal factors relative to the TMD only when signs and symptoms are present. The findings are certainly not conclusive regarding any single factor being consistently associated with a TMD.

The cause of TMD has been considered to be complex and multifactorial. There are numerous factors that can contribute to a TMD. The accepted theory of a multifactorial aetiology of TMD has resulted in a lessening of emphasis on occlusion as the prime aetiological factor. Controlled studies of occlusal factors and TMD show either no relationship or at best only a weak correlation between specific variables and TMD.

A recent systematic review reviewed the literature on the association between features of dental occlusion and temporomandibular disorders and concluded that although there were a few papers that may have suggested a possible association, the existing evidence support the absence of a disease-specific association, and there is no ground to hypothesise a major role for dental occlusion in the pathophysiology of TMDs. They recommended that dental clinicians are encouraged to move forward and abandon the old-fashioned gnathological paradigm.

Further Reading

Al-Ani Z. (2020). Occlusion and Temporomandibular Disorders: A Long-Standing Controversy in Dentistry. *Primary Dental Journal* 9: 43–48.

Burke, F.J., Murray, M.C., and Shortall, A.C. (2005). Trends in indirect dentistry: 6. Provisional restorations, more than just a temporary. *Dent Update* 32: 443–444, 447–8, 450–2.

Egermark-Eriksson, I., Carlsson, G.E., Magnusson, T., and Thilander, B. (1990). A longtudinal study on malocclusion in relation to signs and symptoms of cranio-mandibular disorders in children and adolescents. *Eur J Orthod* 12: 399–407.

Davies, S. (2004). Conformative, re-organized or unorganized? *Dent Update* 31: 334–336, 338–40, 342–5.

Davies, S.J., Gray, R.M., and Smith, P.W. (2001). Good occlusal practice in simple restorative dentistry. *Br Dent J* 191: 365–368, 371–4, 377–81.

Huber, L. and Hall, C. (1990). A comparison of the signs of temporomandibular joint dysfunction and occlusal discrepancies in a symptom-free population of men and women. *Oral Surg Oral Med Oral Pathol* 70: 180–183.

Shargill, I. and Ashley, M. (2006). Good night, squashbite: a 'how to' paper on better wax occlusal records. *Dent Update* 33: 626–628. 631.

Evidence-based Dentistry

Manfredini, D., Lombardo, L., and Siciliani, G. (2017). Temporomandibular disorders and dental occlusion. A systematic review of association studies: end of an era? *J Oral Rehabil* 44: 908–923.

Chapter 9

I've Got Pain in My Face

History

Fiona is a 30-year-old schoolteacher and you have known the family for years. She phones your practice because she is in pain but due to school commitments cannot attend during the day. She is seen by you in your evening emergency space.

She is complaining of pain from her left cheek area. She said the pain began spontaneously about six weeks ago. It was intermittent but is now becoming more frequent. As her students are approaching their GCSE exams, she was busy at school and could not afford time off work to seek advice. Today, however, the pain has become so bad that she can ignore it no longer. She described it as being episodic and sharp, stabbing severe pain that lasts for no more than a few seconds – 'it makes my eyes water!'. It can arise spontaneously, but she notices it more when she washes her face or puts on make-up. She now avoids touching a certain area of her face. She said that she had had similar symptoms about nine months ago which were not as severe and 'went away'. She gets episodes of the sharp pain three or four times a day, but, today, it is much more intense and frequent.

She also has pain brought on by brushing her teeth with cold water and eating cold foods such as ice cream, and her teeth ache for a while after eating or drinking extremes of temperature.

She has not taken any analgesia because she said that she suffers from 'heart-burn'. You have suspected for some time that Fiona is bulimic and you have been concerned about acid erosion of her teeth, particularly on the palatal surfaces of the upper incisors. You have attempted to discuss this with Fiona but she denies making herself sick. About a month ago, you discussed with her the possibility of root canal treatment to an upper left molar tooth because this tooth had become exquisitely sensitive to

Temporomandibular Disorders: A Problem-Based Approach, Second Edition. M. Ziad Al-Ani and Robin J.M. Gray.
© 2021 M. Ziad Al-Ani and Robin J.M. Gray. Published 2021 by John Wiley & Sons Ltd.
Companion Website: www.wiley.com/go/al-ani/temporomandibular-disorders-2e

hot and cold. There was a large area of exposed palatal root of the upper left second molar. She, however, declined because she was too busy and wished to defer any definitive treatment until school broke up for the summer holidays. She said that her symptoms were not exacerbated by stress or by physical activity. Fiona is married; she has two young daughters and lives with them and her husband, who is currently in full-time employment.

She volunteered that she had been to her doctor recently because she feels weepy and stressed. She has the pressure of her job and is also worried about her husband, who is a builder, because she fears that his business is under threat as a result of the economic climate. You have in the past asked her about the erosion on her teeth, but she has consistently denied any untoward habits. You know that she has had a history of increased alcohol intake in the past, but she stopped drinking alcohol when she became pregnant with her first child and has not consumed alcohol since.

She takes thyroxine for an underactive thyroid. She is otherwise fit and well and attends gym classes three evenings a week.

Examination 1

On examination, there was a normal range of mouth movement in the vertical and lateral directions. You examined the temporomandibular joints (TMJs) for tenderness, and there was no tenderness on lateral palpation in the area immediately in front of the ear, on intra-auricular palpation via the external auditory meatus or on manipulation of the mandible to a retruded position. There was intermittent soft clicking in the left TMJ but no crepitation.

She did have signs of parafunction in that she had ridging of the inside of her cheeks and scalloping of the lateral border of her tongue. There was no obvious abnormal wear faceting, and there was no obvious attrition of her teeth. There was, however, erosion of the enamel on the palatal surfaces of her upper teeth, especially the incisors and molars. The palatal root of the upper left second molar was exposed, and there was approximately 7 mm of gingival recession. There was no masticatory muscle tenderness. You examined the masseter and temporalis muscles by digital palpation and you examined the lateral pterygoid against resistance.

When you examined her occlusion she appeared to have centric relation occlusion; there was no premature contact, and there was no slide from centric relation to centric occlusion. On lateral excursions of the mandible, she had canine guidance, and there were no obvious interferences on the working or non-working side. She had good oral hygiene; there were no calculus or plaque deposits. She had heavily restored posterior teeth, but no teeth were tender to percussion, although she said that the upper left second molar felt 'slightly different'. She had generalised sensitivity due to gingival recession and the erosion on the palatal surfaces of her upper teeth; this was particularly noticeable around the region of the upper left first molar.

Radiographic examination

In view of the fact that she had heavily filled posterior teeth and because you had not taken bite-wing radiographs for about 18 months, you took right and left bite-wing radiographs and a periapical of UL7 at the time of her examination. These radiographs showed her restorations to be in good condition. There was no primary or recurrent caries and no apical pathology. There were no obvious deposits of calculus and the bone level appeared normal apart from the upper left quadrant where there was slight horizontal bone loss.

Differential diagnosis

 Tunnel vision is dangerous. It is your responsibility when diagnosing a patient with a history of facial pain to consider all possibilities.

Dental practitioners should try to identify the underlying mechanisms of pain in the orofacial region for all of their patients. Pain in the jaw joint and muscles is not always due to simple nociceptive pain mechanisms but may involve inflammatory, neuropathic and functional components. While it may be more common to see nociceptive and inflammatory types of pain in the TMJ region, clinicians should consider the possibility of other types of pain in this region, because it will influence the management strategy as well as the eventual outcome.

The International Classification of Orofacial Pain (ICOP) 2020 gives six primary classifications, each with multiple subdivisions:

1. **Orofacial pain attributed to disorders of dentoalveolar and anatomically related structures**
   1.1 Dental pain
       1.1.1 Pulpal pain
       1.1.2 Periodontal pain
       1.1.3 Gingival pain
   1.2 Oral mucosal, salivary gland, and jaw bone pains
       1.2.1 Oral mucosal pain
       1.2.2 Salivary gland pain
       1.2.3 Jaw bone pain
2. **Myofascial orofacial pain**
   2.1 Primary myofascial orofacial pain
       2.1.1 Acute primary myofascial orofacial pain
       2.1.2 Chronic primary myofascial orofacial pain
   2.2 Secondary myofascial orofacial pain
       2.2.1 Myofascial orofacial pain attributed to tendonitis

2.2.2 Myofascial orofacial pain attributed to myositis

2.2.3 Myofascial orofacial pain attributed to muscle spasm

3. **TMJ pain**

   3.1 Primary temporomandibular joint pain

      3.1.1 Acute primary temporomandibular joint pain

      3.1.2 Chronic primary temporomandibular joint pain

   3.2 Secondary temporomandibular joint pain

      3.2.1 Temporomandibular joint pain attributed to arthritis

      3.2.2 Temporomandibular joint pain attributed to disc displacement

      3.2.3 Temporomandibular joint pain attributed to degenerative joint disease

      3.2.4 Temporomandibular joint pain attributed to subluxation

4. **Orofacial pain attributed to lesion or disease of the cranial nerves**

   4.1 Pain attributed to lesion or disease of the trigeminal nerve

      4.1.1 Trigeminal neuralgia

      4.1.2 Other trigeminal neuropathic pain

   4.2 Pain attributed to lesion or disease of the glossopharyngeal nerve

      4.2.1 Glossopharyngeal neuralgia

      4.2.2 Glossopharyngeal neuropathic pain

5. **Orofacial pains resembling presentations of primary headaches**

   5.1 Orofacial migraine

      5.1.1 Episodic orofacial migraine

      5.1.2 Chronic orofacial migraine

   5.2 Tension-type orofacial pain

   5.3 Trigeminal autonomic orofacial pain

      5.3.1 Orofacial cluster attacks

      5.3.2 Paroxysmal hemifacial pain

      5.3.3 Short-lasting unilateral neuralgiform facial pain attacks with cranial autonomic symptoms (SUNFA)

      5.3.4 Hemifacial continuous pain with autonomic symptoms

   5.4 Neurovascular orofacial pain

      5.4.1 Short-lasting neurovascular orofacial pain

      5.4.2 Long-lasting neurovascular orofacial pain

6. **Idiopathic orofacial pain**

   6.1 Burning mouth syndrome (BMS)

      6.1.1 BMS without somatosensory changes

      6.1.2 BMS with somatosensory changes

      6.1.3 Probable BMS

   6.2 Persistent idiopathic facial pain

      6.2.1 Persistent idiopathic facial pain without somatosensory changes

      6.2.2 Persistent idiopathic facial pain with somatosensory changes

      6.2.3 Probable persistent idiopathic facial pain

   6.3 Persistent idiopathic dentoalveolar pain

      6.3.1 Persistent idiopathic dentoalveolar pain without somatosensory changes

6.3.2 Persistent idiopathic dentoalveolar pain with somatosensory changes

6.3.3 Probable persistent idiopathic dentoalveolar pain

6.4 Constant unilateral facial pain with additional attacks (CUFPA)

Let us consider all possible sources of Fiona's symptoms:

- Dental (pulpitis, pericoronitis, and apical periodontitis)
- Fractured tooth
- Temporomandibular disorder (TMD)
- Neuralgic pain
- Sinus pain
- Ear infection
- Headache
- Soft tissue
- Cervical spine pain
- Salivary glands
- Atypical facial pain
- Referred cardiac pain
- Multiple sclerosis
- Central lesion
- Tumour (acoustic neuroma)
- Ophthalmic
- Dry socket
- Trauma

Let us deal with the list in reverse order.

 It should be possible to eliminate most of these potential diagnoses by history taking and discussion. Her symptoms are too specific for them to be coming from an ophthalmic problem, although if you have any doubt you should suggest that she sees her optician to have her eyesight tested.

 Dry socket and trauma can be immediately excluded in the absence of any germane history of either a blow or a recent dental extraction.

Had there been a central lesion or an acoustic neuroma, you would have expected other symptoms such as possible involvement of the cranial nerves and headache or continual facial pain. You thought about a tumour such as an acoustic neuroma, but this would, however, have been accompanied by an alteration to her hearing.

 Multiple sclerosis on rare occasions presents with facial pain but should be remembered because, on occasion, the first symptoms can mimic the distribution of pain found in patients with a TMD and on rare occasions can occur before any other signs such as muscle wasting or weakness. This is extremely rare and normally accompanied by other symptoms.

 If her pain had been referred as cardiac pain, this would have been expected over the area of her left mandible, in her left arm and the left side of her neck. This would have been possible if her pain had been anginal in origin. She did state, however, that her symptoms were not worse with stress or physical activity, and she is a regular fitness participant.

 She may have atypical facial pain, but this is also highly unlikely because true atypical facial pain tends to be bizarre in its pain pattern and presentation. It does not tend to localise to one particular area and frequently crosses the midline. A diagnosis of atypical facial pain is very rare.

 If her symptoms had arisen from her salivary glands, you would have expected her to suffer intense pain at mealtimes when the salivary flow is stimulated. This is often accompanied by localised swelling over the parotid or submandibular glands. The pain and swelling would subsequently gradually resolve unless there was infection in the gland. There would then be other symptoms such as very painful localised swelling and a bad taste.

 Referred cervical spine pain from the C5 and C6 level can present as facial pain but this is most commonly over the angle of the mandible, not the maxilla, because this distribution follows neural pathways. There is sometimes a history of a previous neck injury. If there had been pain from the cervical spine, this would have been associated with other symptoms such as restricted movement and acute localised tenderness. If you are in any doubt, however, you should refer her to a neurologist directly or via her general medical practitioner.

 If there had been a soft-tissue lesion, such as a large aphthous or traumatic ulcer, you would have been able to visualise this.

 Headache, commonly migraine, can present with unusual symptoms. These usually involve nausea and sometimes vomiting, a visual aura, and photophobia. There is frequently a family history. You should be able to eliminate this diagnosis from Fiona's history especially as there is not a specific trigger for headache arising from touch.

 If Fiona had had an ear infection, she would have probably had a discharge from her ear canal or the inner aspect of the external auditory meatus would have been very tender to touch, and the tympanic membrane would have been tender and swollen.

 Having considered the possible diagnoses and eliminated the impossible and unlikely, let us revisit the original list of possibilities and see what remains:

- Dental (pulpitis, pericoronitis, and apical periodontitis)
- Neuralgic pain
- Fractured tooth
- TMD
- Sinus pain

You should be able to eliminate any problems from her sinuses. If she had sinusitis, the pain would be worse when she lay down at night or when she bent forward to pick something up from the floor. There is a gravitational influence in sinusitis, and if there is a fluid level in the sinus when the patient bends forward pain becomes much more intense. The area underneath the zygoma is often tender to palpate. The eye on the affected side can become bloodshot and watery. There is sometimes a bad taste in the mouth and patients usually describe a 'heavy feeling' on the affected side of the face. Even if there is no fluid level in the sinus, mucosal thickening can cause similar symptoms.

In her case a TMD is highly unlikely. Fiona did have an intermittent click, but this was totally symptomless and occasional. It had never caused pain and she had never experienced locking. She had no muscle tenderness or TMJ tenderness and her range of jaw movement was normal. Clicking on its own is not considered to be diagnostic of a TMD.

A hairline fracture in a tooth is a possibility, but you would expect this to be accompanied by part of the tooth in question being tender when placed under pressure. The tooth is usually very easily identified because, when biting pressure is applied, the patient will feel a sharp acute pain in the tooth. This can usually be diagnosed by applying pressure to each of the cusps in turn, or asking the patient to bite down hard on a cotton-wool roll. On occasion, it may be necessary to remove any restoration in the tooth and flex the cusps to determine whether or not there is a hairline fracture. These fractures are sometimes very difficult if not impossible to visualise or detect on radiographic examination.

This leaves us with two possible diagnoses:

- Dental pain (pulpitis, pericoronitis, and apical periodontitis)
- Neuralgic pain.

When considering dental pain excluding a cuspal fracture, there are three possible diagnoses: pulpitis, pericoronitis, and apical periodontitis.

Pericoronitis can be eliminated if there is no obvious evidence of infection, restricted opening, or direct tenderness of the soft tissues, usually around the upper or lower third molar. Any of these symptoms would be detectable visually. She might also experience a bad taste or halitosis.

There was a large area of exposed palatal root on the upper left second molar and you felt that a terminal pulpitis was developing. You had discussed this with her some time previously, but her symptoms in relation to this particular tooth had not worsened since. Although she did volunteer that this tooth 'felt different', it was not tender to percussion.

Apical periodontitis is therefore at this stage unlikely but irreversible pulpitis is a distinct diagnostic possibility. You had discussed the possibility of root canal treatment to the upper left second molar with Fiona, and you agreed that this would need to be done soon because you felt that the nerve was dying. Some elements of the history are not suggestive of this being the sole cause of her symptoms, however. If she had pulpitis, you would have expected sharp pain in response to a stimulus or arising spontaneously with dull pain lasting for some time thereafter. The same is true of extreme dentine sensitivity.

Having logically eliminated all other possible diagnoses, you are left with one that you felt was most likely.

Neuralgic pain

You reviewed her history, and she said that she had episodes of being completely pain-free, but then she experienced sudden, sharp episodes of severe pain, which was enough to 'stop me in my tracks'. The pain made her eye water and was severe. She found it occurred spontaneously or when she applied make-up over the left side of her face and when she washed her face. You had examined all other aspects of her articulatory system and found no conclusive signs or symptoms.

Your final diagnosis therefore was one of trigeminal neuralgia. This is usually described by patients as being a short, sharp, shooting pain that lasts for seconds and is severe. The pain then disappears and in-between times there are no other symptoms. This can arise spontaneously without any initiating factor. It is possible for trigeminal neuralgia to 'burn out' in the fullness of time. This diagnosis is compatible with the fact that she experienced a similar episode that resolved spontaneously some months ago.

Treatment

Dentists can prescribe the drug used in the management of trigeminal neuralgia – carbamazepine (Tegretol). Even if you are experienced in management of this condition, treatment should always be undertaken by the patient's general medical practitioner. The first line of treatment is carbamazepine starting at a dose of 100 mg twice a day. This dose is usually increased to 200 mg three times a day. It should be remembered in this case, however, that there was a previous history of increased alcohol intake. This may have led to some liver damage. A liver function test should be carried out before prescription and at regular intervals, subsequently.

She is taking thyroxine; metabolism of this is accelerated by carbamazepine so her dose of thyroxine may need to be increased. In view of this, it would be essential for you to refer her to her general medical practitioner for her treatment and subsequent monitoring.

When carbamazepine is prescribed patients must be warned of possible side effects such as fever, sore throat, rash, mouth ulcers and bruising. Once a maintenance dose has been achieved, it is normal to gradually reduce this in an attempt to wean the patient off prescription when clinically advisable.

In Fiona's case, you conducted an exhaustive examination of all possible structures involved. In view of the absence of any clinical or radiographic findings, and in view of her specific history, you diagnosed trigeminal neuralgia.

After receiving a letter from you, Fiona's doctor commenced a course of Tegretol. She had regular monitoring and her treatment proceeded uneventfully. After three months of increasing her medication, her doctor started to reduce the dose, and she was weaned off all treatment nine months later. She is now symptom-free. In the meantime, you undertook root canal therapy to the upper left second molar.

Questions to ask patients regarding pain in general

Site

- Where do you feel the pain?
- Can you locate the pain?
- Does the pain radiate anywhere else or even across the midline?

Character

- Is the pain throbbing, stabbing, or shooting? Pain can range from being a dull ache to severe shooting pain.

Severity

- How bad is the pain on a scale of 1–10?
- Has the pain got worse since it started?
- Has the pain got less since it started?
- Do you have to take painkillers – if so, what?
- Does the pain wake you up at night?

Duration and frequency

- Does the pain remain for a long time or does it go in a matter of seconds?
- Is the pain intermittent?
- Does it come and go on an hourly, daily or weekly basis?
- How long have you had it?

Onset and time

- When did you first notice the pain?
- Is there any particular time of day when you notice the pain?
- Is it worse in the morning, easing off during the day, or are you pain free in the morning and the pain gets worse during the day?
- Can you associate the onset of symptoms with a specific event?
- Does anything trigger the pain such as touching an area of your face, shaving or putting on makeup?
- Are there exacerbating or relieving factors?
- Is the pain related to eating? Association with mealtimes can indicate several possible diagnoses such as hot or cold foods or sugary foods causing pulpal pain, movement of the mandible causing muscle pain, and sialadenitis causing pain from the salivary glands.
- Is the pain bought on by biting?
- Do you notice if the pain is related to lying down or bending down?

- Is there anything that makes the pain better or worse?
- Does the pain start with hot or cold stimulus?
- What have you tried for pain relief?
- Have you attended your dentist or your doctor with this problem before?
- Have you been prescribed any drugs for the pain?
- Do you feel that your pain is stress related?

Generally, **SOCRATES** is a mnemonic acronym which can be used to evaluate the nature of pain that a patient is experiencing.

- Site
- Onset
- Character
- Radiation
- Associations
- Time course
- Exacerbating/relieving factors
- Severity

Further Reading

Barnes, M.F., Geary, J.L., Clifford, T.J., and Lamey, P.J. (2006). Fitting acrylic occlusal splints and an experimental laminated appliance used in migraine prevention therapy. *Br Dent J* 200: 283–286. discussion 269.

Cadden, S.W. and Orchardson, R. (2001). The neural mechanisms of oral and facial pain. *Dent Update* 28: 359–367.

Glaros, A.G. (2008). Temporomandibular disorders and facial pain: a psychophysiological perspective. *Appl Psychophysiol Biofeedback* 33: 161–171.

(2020). International Classification of Orofacial Pain, 1st edition (ICOP). *Cephalalgia* 40: 129–221.

Jorns, T.P. and Zakrzewska, J.M. (2007). Evidence-based approach to the medical management of trigeminal neuralgia. *Br J Neurosurg* 21 (3): 253–261.

Madland, G., Newton-John, T., and Feinmann, C. (2001). Chronic idiopathic orofacial pain: I: what is the evidence base? *Br Dent J* 191: 22–24.

Newton-John, T., Madland, G., and Feinmann, C. (2001). Chronic idiopathic orofacial pain: II. What can the general dental practitioner do? *Br Dent J* 191: 72–73.

Prasad, S. and Galetta, S. (2009). Trigeminal neuralgia: historical notes and current concepts. *Neurologist* 15: 87–94.

Scully, C. and Felix, D.H. (2006). Oral medicine–update for the dental practitioner orofacial pain. *Br Dent J* 200: 75–83.

Svensson, P. and Baad-Hansen, L. (2010). The mechanisms of joint and muscle pain. *J Am Dent Assoc* 141: 672–674.

Van Kleef, M., van Genderen, W.E., Narouze, S. et al. (2009). 1. Trigeminal neuralgia. *Pain Pract* 9: 252–259.

Zakrzewska, J.M. (2007). Diagnosis and management of non-dental orofacial pain. *Dent Update* 34: 134–136. 138–9.

Zakrzewska JM, Linskey ME. Trigeminal neuralgia. *Clin Evid (Online)* 2009. Available at: http://clinicalevidence.bmj.com/ceweb/conditions/nud/1207/1207_I14.jsp (accessed October 2010).

Zakrzewska JM. Differential diagnosis of facial pain and guidelines for management. *Br J Anaesth*. 2013 Jul; 111(1): 95–104.

Chapter 10

I've Got a Dislocated Jaw

You are on call one weekend when your on-call mobile phone rings, and you are requested to re-attend and reopen your surgery urgently. You are advised by the wife of one of your patients that he has been struck in the face playing football, and he cannot close his mouth. She said he has got 'lock jaw'. She says that she is on her way to the surgery and will meet you there.

As you re-attend the practice, your patient and his wife are driving into the car park. He is still dressed in his football kit and is in obvious pain. He is holding a towel to his mouth as he is dribbling saliva. There is no bleeding.

You reopen the surgery and with the assistance of his wife take a history. It would appear that Steven had been trying to head the ball. He had leapt up but had clashed heads with a defender. He remembers that he had his mouth open at the time and the defender's head hit him on the right side of his chin. He was stunned but not rendered unconscious and fell to the ground. He was immediately aware of acute pain in both right and left temporomandibular joints (TMJ)s and also aware that he could not close his mouth. He felt that any attempt at jaw movement was acutely painful. He was also aware of the fact that his mandible had slewed across to the left side and that a depression had appeared in front of his right ear.

It was apparent during history taking that he could not speak comfortably or clearly and was relying on writing notes and his wife interpreting his account of events. He was also not able to swallow comfortably and was dribbling saliva. He was in obvious and increasing pain and his wife estimated that it was less than half an hour since the trauma occurred. Steven and his family were new patients to your practice and you had only seen him once before. He had no relevant medical history and he had a restoration and caries-free mouth. His oral hygiene was excellent.

Temporomandibular Disorders: A Problem-Based Approach, Second Edition. M. Ziad Al-Ani and Robin J.M. Gray.
© 2021 M. Ziad Al-Ani and Robin J.M. Gray. Published 2021 by John Wiley & Sons Ltd.
Companion Website: www.wiley.com/go/al-ani/temporomandibular-disorders-2e

Examination 1

On extraoral examination, there were no contusions, abrasions, or lacerations on Steven's face. There was, however, a red area over the body of the mandible, in the canine region on the right side, and this would appear to correspond with the area that his opponent's head struck. Steven's mouth was stuck open at approximately 25 mm. When being asked to move his mandible, any movement was obviously painful, and he could move to increase his opening by only 3 or 4 mm. He was unable to close his mouth any further and lateral movements were too painful for him to perform, although he did volunteer that even if the pain had not been there, he didn't think he would be able to move his jaw sideways. His chin was obviously deviated to the left side.

Examination of the origin of the masseter muscles was extremely uncomfortable and you were not sure whether you were eliciting pain from the muscle itself or by palpating in the area around the TMJs. There was temporalis tenderness of the vertical fibres in the anterior part of the temple on the right side. Tenderness was also apparent on the left side but less so. You were unable to examine the lateral pterygoid muscles against resistance because he could not stand any pressure under his chin as a result of pain and could not exert any lateral pressure.

Radiographs

You had facilities to take only intraoral radiographs but could not do this because he could neither open nor close his mouth. In addition, you decided that these would be of no diagnostic value.

Other special tests

 You did feel that an extra oral radiograph of his TMJs such as a transcranial oblique lateral (TOL) view would be of value, but the practice that you normally refer your patients to for extraoral radiographs was closed, and there was no local hospital near enough for you to refer him.

Likely diagnoses

 You felt that there were three possible diagnoses: first he had suffered an acute disc displacement because of the trauma to his jaw, and this was what was severely limiting his mouth movement; an alternative diagnosis was that he had fractured his jaw; and the third diagnosis was that he had in fact dislocated his mandible.

 If he had suffered an acute disc displacement, the diagnosis would be one of an internal derangement of his right TMJ with acute disc displacement without reduction. The clinical features of this would, however, have been different from his presentation. In acute disc displacement, he would not have been able to open his mouth beyond 17–20 mm, but he would have been able to close it. He may not have been able to approximate his teeth completely because, if there is acute disc displacement, the highly innervated posterior bilaminar zone can become interposed between the head of the condyle and the glenoid fossa. This means that, although he could almost bring his teeth together, to completely approximate the molar teeth on the affected side would probably cause sharp pain within the TMJ. A degree of mandibular movement would, however, have been possible. He would have felt that he could open his mouth to a certain stage, but at that point, there was a physical obstruction to further movement.

 If he had fractured his mandible, there would have been facial swelling and possibly intraoral bleeding or a haematoma. He would have a degree of jaw movement even though this would have been painful. You would probably have been able to move the fractured parts of the mandible. There might have been a step in the occlusal plane, and he might have had paraesthesia in the distribution of the mental nerve.

 As this patient could neither open nor close his mouth, coupled with the fact that the mandible was slewed across towards the left side, the correct diagnosis, even without radiographs, would be a unilateral dislocation of the mandible on the right side. Had you had the opportunity to take extraoral radiographs, these would have been taken only to confirm your diagnosis because this condition should be readily diagnosed on clinical evidence alone, and this would not have been sufficient reason for taking them. A TOL radiograph would have shown the glenoid fossa on the right side to be empty, and the head of the condyle to be displaced forwards and upwards well in advance of the articular eminence. This would have been less obvious on a dental panoramic tomogram (DPT) which would have been very difficult to take because he could not close to bite on the spacer.

 What happens in dislocation is that the mandible is struck, usually with the mouth open. The head of the condyle is displaced anterior to the eminence and then muscle spasm occurs and the pull of the masseter and temporalis impacts the head of the condyle against the articular eminence preventing the condyle slipping back into place (Figures 10.1 and 10.2).

Management

 When dislocation of the mandible occurs, the sooner the dislocation is reduced, the easier it is to do. If the mandible has been dislocated for several hours, it is often very difficult if not impossible to reposition and, on occasions such as this, the patient should be referred to your local hospital accident and emergency department (A&E), where the dislocation can be reduced usually with the use of intravenous sedation such as midazolam.

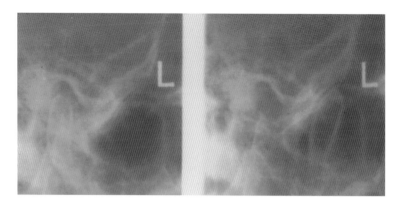

Figure 10.1 Transcranial oblique lateral (closed and open) radiographs showing an empty fossa with the head of the condyle displaced anterior and superior to the articular eminence in TMJ dislocation. (M. Ziad Al-Ani, Robin J.M. Gray.)

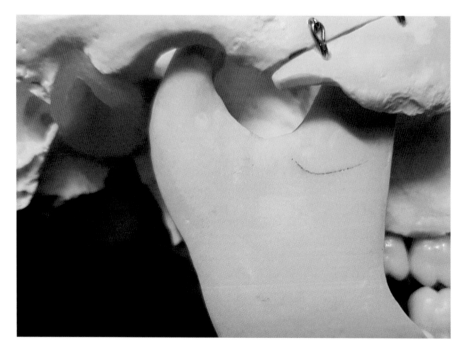

Figure 10.2 In dislocation, the head of the condyle is displaced anterior to the eminence. (M. Ziad Al-Ani, Robin J.M. Gray.)

 If the situation is dealt with quickly, however, it is often possible to manually reduce the dislocation at the chair side. There are two methods of doing this: first by wrapping gauze around the operator's thumbs and placing the thumbs on the molar teeth, then applying firm pressure downwards and posteriorly on the affected side while attempting to 'distract' the head of the condyle (Figure 10.3a,b). This method is successful on

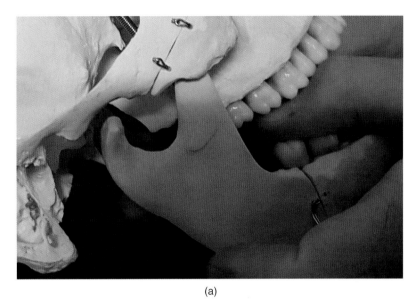

(a)

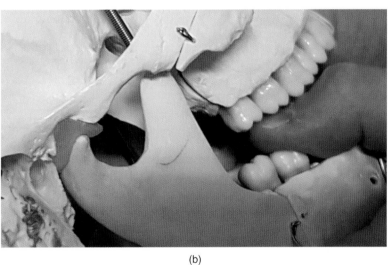

(b)

Figure 10.3 (a) Manually reducing the dislocation by placing the operator's thumbs on the molar teeth, then applying firm pressure downwards and posteriorly on the affected side. (b) The head of the condyle is slipped back into place. (M. Ziad Al-Ani, Robin J.M. Gray.)

occasions, but there is often subconscious tensing of the muscles by the patient, or alternatively, the sudden downward pressure induces intense muscle spasm, rendering reduction of the dislocation impossible.

An alternative method is to hold the mandible firmly yet gently in the midline region with one finger inside the mouth and the other fingers under the chin, and in the molar region on the affected side with one finger again on the surface of the molar teeth and the other fingers under the body of the mandible. The mandible is then gently manipulated up and down in a 'jiggling' fashion with gentle distal and downward pressure being applied on the affected side. With this method, it is not unusual for the condyle to slip back into place, but often, only after performing this manipulation for up to a minute or two. The muscles will gradually relax, allowing the head of the condyle to slip back into place. This is the preferred method to try in the first instance.

If reduction is unsuccessful, prompt referral to the nearest hospital A&E is advised. If reduction is successful, the patient should be counselled because his TMJ and muscles will remain painful for two to three days. He should be advised to take non-steroidal anti-inflammatory drugs as long as there are no medical contraindications to doing this. He should be advised to stick rigidly to a soft diet and give his TMJ as much chance to rest as possible and should be warned to strictly limit mouth opening.

When dislocation of the mandible occurs in a situation such as this, it is usually a 'one-off' situation and recurrent dislocation does not become a problem.

If a patient has recurrent dislocation of the mandible that is unrelated to trauma, and if conservative measures have failed, the patient cannot self-reduce the dislocation and, if the situation is unacceptable, the treatment is usually surgical.

The joint can be injected with a mild sclerosing solution in an attempt to artificially induce adhesions within the joint, thereby limiting the range of movement.

Invasive intracapsular surgical procedures include eminectomy. This is a surgical procedure in which the articular eminence is flattened or surgically reduced, allowing the head of the condyle free movement; however, as the eminence has been removed the head of the condyle will not impact, thereby preventing it slipping back into place.

Alternatively, a procedure can be undertaken to increase the height of the articular eminence (Dautrey's procedure), thereby producing a physical block to the condyle and preventing it dislocating in the first place.

It should be noted, however, that a procedure such as this will limit the normal range of mandibular movement on a permanent basis.

Recently autologous blood injection has been suggested as a possible treatment of chronic recurrent TMJ dislocation. Some authors believe that this technique may create a bed for fibrous tissue formation in the TMJ area, which may lead to formation of adhesion in the joint space causing a restriction of mandibular movement.

A recent systematic review investigated the use of autologous blood injection for treatment of chronic recurrent TMJ dislocation and found that there are a few studies about this technique and although there were some successful results about this modality reported in these studies, some concerns, however, are still there about the effect of the injected blood on the articular cartilage and formation of fibrous or bony ankylosis. The authors of this review suggested that the long-term mouth opening is not known and serial injections with immobilization may be needed.

Further Reading

Baur, D.A., Jannuzzi, J.R., Mercan, U., and Quereshy, F.A. (2013). Treatment of long term anterior dislocation of the TMJ. *Int J Oral Maxillofac Surg* 42: 1030–1033.

Caminiti, M.F. and Weinberg, S. (1998). Chronic mandibular dislocation: the role of non-surgical and surgical treatment. *J Can Dent Assoc* 64: 484–491.

Guarda-Nardini, L., Palumbo, B., Manfredini, D., and Ferronato, G. (2008). Surgical treatment of chronic temporomandibular joint dislocation: a case report. *Oral Maxillofac Surg* 12: 43–46.

Guven, O. (2009). Management of chronic recurrent temporomandibular joint dislocations: a retrospective study. *J Craniomaxillofac Surg* 37: 24–29.

Liddell, A. and Perez, D.E. (2015). Temporomandibular joint dislocation. *Oral Maxillofac Surg Clin North Am* 27: 125–136.

Martins, W.D., Ribas Mde, O., Bisinelli, J. et al. (2014). Recurrent dislocation of the temporomandibular joint: a literature review and two case reports treated with eminectomy. *Cranio* 32: 110–117.

Mustafa el, M. and Sidebottom, A. (2014). Risk factors for intraoperative dislocation of the total temporomandibular joint replacement and its management. *Br J Oral Maxillofac Surg* 52: 190–192.

Ogawa, M., Kanbe, T., Kano, A. et al. (2015). Conservative reduction by lever action of chronic bilateral mandibular condyle dislocation. *Cranio* 33: 142–147.

Okamoto, T., Kaibuchi, N., Sasaki, R. et al. (2020). Eminectomy with restraint of the joint capsule to treat chronic and recurrent dislocation of the temporomandibular joint. *Br J Oral Maxillofac Surg* 58: 366–368.

Pradhan, L., Jaisani, M.R., Sagtani, A., and Win, A. (2015). Conservative management of chronic TMJ dislocation: an old technique revived. *J Maxillofac Oral Surg* 14 (Suppl 1): 267–270.

Sharma, N.K., Singh, A.K., Pandey, A. et al. (2015). Temporomandibular joint dislocation. *Natl J Maxillofac Surg* 6: 16–20.

Stembirek, J., Matalova, E., Buchtova, M. et al. (2013). Investigation of an autologous blood treatment strategy for temporomandibular joint hypermobility in a pig model. *Int J Oral Maxillofac Surg* 42: 369–375.

Evidence-based Dentistry

Varedi, P. and Bohluli, B. (2015). Autologous blood injection for treatment of chronic recurrent TMJ dislocation: is it successful? Is it safe enough? A systematic review [published correction appears in Oral Maxillofac Surg. 2015 Sep;19(3):329-31]. *Oral Maxillofac Surg* 19: 243–252.

Chapter 11

My Teeth Are Worn

History

Jonathan is a 48-year-old barrister. He has a very busy, pressurised, and stressful job. He is not a regular dental attender because he finds it very difficult to set aside time for routine appointments and tends to come in for advice only when he has a problem. He is very conscious of his appearance because he spends a lot of time in court and feels that he is 'on show'. Over the last two to three years, he has been very conscious of the fact that his teeth are wearing. He thinks that the appearance of his teeth is embarrassing and is also aware of the fact that the lower third of his face feels over-closed. He was conscious of wear of his upper and lower incisor teeth.

He has generalised sensitivity to sweet and cold, and he has recently lost two mesioincisal restorations in his upper central incisors. This has prompted him to seek treatment today. He said that he started noticing wear in his teeth about six or seven years ago, and it has become much worse over the last two to three years.

There is no adverse medical history, he is not under the care of his doctor, and he takes no medication. There is no history of gastric reflux or of vomiting. He is a smoker and a fairly heavy drinker consuming 35+ units of alcohol per week.

He has no history of facial pain but did volunteer that he got occasional discomfort from his left jaw joint and from the left side of his face. He said he thought that his bite had altered. He did not know whether or not he ground or clenched his teeth, but he suspected that he did not because his wife had never told him that she had been disturbed by him doing this at night. You asked if he would be interested in keeping a diet sheet, but he was resistant of this idea and told you with some impatience that

Temporomandibular Disorders: A Problem-Based Approach, Second Edition. M. Ziad Al-Ani and Robin J.M. Gray.
© 2021 M. Ziad Al-Ani and Robin J.M. Gray. Published 2021 by John Wiley & Sons Ltd.
Companion Website: www.wiley.com/go/al-ani/temporomandibular-disorders-2e

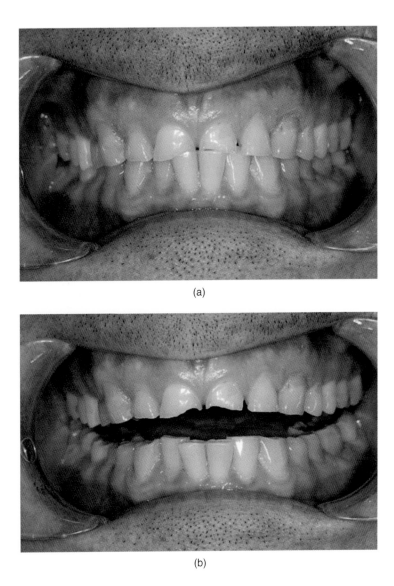

(a)

(b)

Figure 11.1 Gross tooth surface loss secondary to parafunction. (M. Ziad Al-Ani, Robin J.M. Gray.)

he had 'no time for that sort of thing'. His concerns were solely aesthetic (Figure 11.1).

Examination 1

Jonathan has an Angle's class I, basal bone and incisal relationship. He has a normal range of mouth opening in the vertical and lateral dimensions, being able to open to 47 mm vertically and to move his mandible 12 mm to both the right and the left sides. When you examined the pathway of

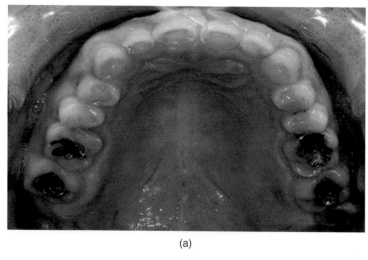

(a)

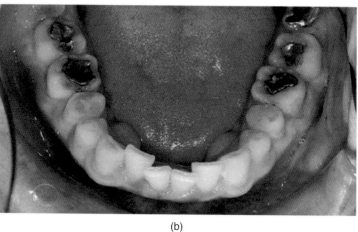

(b)

Figure 11.2 Occlusal views showing marked tooth surface loss, exposed dentine and worn restorations. (M. Ziad Al-Ani, Robin J.M. Gray.)

opening, this was straight, indicating that both joints were working synchronously. There were no joint sounds, neither clicking nor crepitation. On examination intraorally you noticed very marked ridging of the buccal mucosa on both the right and the left sides, and there was obvious scalloping of the lateral border of the tongue. There was marked attrition involving upper and lower anterior teeth, the canines and the molar teeth, where enamel had been lost to the extent that the dentine was exposed (Figure 11.2). He appeared over-closed with a free-way space that you estimated to be about 5 mm.

On examination of the temporomandibular joints (TMJs), the left TMJ was tender on lateral and intra-auricular palpation, and the left masseter and temporalis muscles were tender to palpate but only mildly so.

On examination of the occlusion, centric relation and centric occlusion did not coincide, the premature contact being between the upper left second premolar and the lower left first molar. The slide from centric relation to centric occlusion was vertical and to the left and was marked in both dimensions.

On examination of the soft tissues, the BPE in all six sextants surprisingly was three, although his oral hygiene appeared satisfactory.

On examination of the teeth, there was generalised tooth surface loss. Mesial incisal bonded composite restorations had been lost from both upper central incisors.

You got the impression that this patient was not particularly interested in his overall dental condition or the causative factors of his toothwear. What he was interested in was an aesthetic 'makeover' to improve the appearance of his teeth, and for you to do something about his perceived loss in vertical height in the lower third of his face, thereby restoring his facial contours.

Radiographic examination (Bitewings)

Radiographic examination showed there to be no primary or recurrent caries, but there was evidence of early horizontal bone loss in all four quadrants.

Diagnosis

When considering your diagnosis, you felt that it was important to discuss the possible causes of tooth surface loss. Despite the multifactoral aetiology of tooth surface loss, certain clinical features may suggest that the major contributory factor to surface loss could be due to acid attack on dentine (erosion). When erosion affects the palatal surfaces of upper maxillary teeth, there is often a central area of exposed dentine surrounded by a border of unaffected enamel (cupping).

In view of the fact that he had all the clinical signs of a parafunctional activity, such as bruxism or tooth clenching, and in view of his occlusal discrepancies, you felt that his tooth surface loss was secondary to parafunctional activity.

Treatment

Your initial advice was to suggest construction of an occlusally balanced centric relation stabilisation splint. This would have two functions: first of all, to act as a habit breaker to discourage his parafunctional activity and prevent further damage to his teeth and, second, as a diagnostic measure to try to establish an increased vertical height with which he would be comfortable. This would give you some treatment plan for working towards restoration of his occlusion.

He refused this treatment suggestion and, on reflection, you realised that he would not wear a splint even if it were provided for him.

You discussed his diet and, although he would not commit to completing a diet sheet, he said that he drank very few acidic drinks but did admit to consuming over five units of alcohol a day on average. He did not drink fizzy drinks. Other possible intrinsic causes of erosion include reflux and vomiting but he denied this.

In view of the complexity of his treatment, his high demands and the fact that he would not wear a stabilisation splint, you would not have been able to confirm an acceptable increase in vertical dimension.

You therefore referred him to a specialist in fixed and removable prosthodontics for a definitive treatment plan.

The specialist advised you that his plan would involve mounting models on a semi-adjustable articulator in centric jaw relation and undertaking a diagnostic wax-up to determine the occlusal plane, the aesthetics and the increased vertical dimension that would be determined by the first contact in centric relation (in his case the UL5/LL6). A template would then be fabricated, and the new restorations could be completed to this reorganised occlusion and the posterior interferences eliminated. The specialist went to great lengths to explain these steps in detail, adding that this would be a long course of treatment and, once started, would have to be completed. The patient accepted this and was pleased that he would notice an immediate improvement in aesthetics once the provisional restorations were placed at the increased vertical dimension. The provisional restorations would be replaced in sequence as the permanent restorations were fitted (Figure 11.3).

Important considerations in tooth surface loss

Abrasion

Abrasion is wear of the teeth by surfaces other than teeth, e.g. a toothbrush. Cervical lesions caused purely by abrasion have sharply defined margins and a smooth hard surface. The lesion may become more rounded and shallow if there is an element of erosion present (Figure 11.4).

Attrition

Attrition results from tooth-to-tooth contact which produces well-defined wear facets on the functional surfaces of the teeth that match corresponding lesions on the teeth in the opposing jaw. If wear is primarily attritional, dentine tends to wear at the same rate as the surrounding enamel. The wear is usually uniform when opposing teeth are affected. Flattening of cusps or incisal edges and localised facets on occlusal or palatal surfaces would indicate a primary attritional aetiology. With improved life

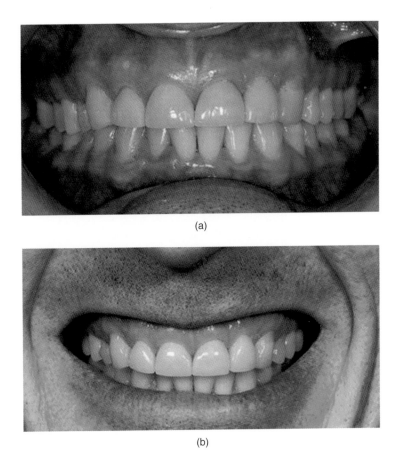

(a)

(b)

Figure 11.3 Restored occlusion. (M. Ziad Al-Ani, Robin J.M. Gray.)

expectancy and control of dental caries and periodontal disease, it is likely that retention of natural teeth into older age will lead to a higher prevalence of worn dentition as a result of attrition (Figure 11.5), although this is not the case with your patient.

Parafunction

Parafunctional habits, such as bruxism and clenching, are believed to be important factors in causing accelerated attrition. If bruxism is severe either marked wear of occlusal surfaces will occur or, in cases of compromised periodontal support, tooth mobility may result. Bruxism can also be associated with muscle pain, fractured teeth and restorations, and tooth sensitivity (Figure 11.6).

Tooth surface loss or tooth wear cannot be taken as a sign that the patient is actively bruxing. Even if the cause of the tooth surface loss was bruxism, the patient may no longer have active parafunction. Tooth sensitivity is a common symptom and repeated tooth or restoration fracture or failure is often reported. The two most reliable signs of active bruxism

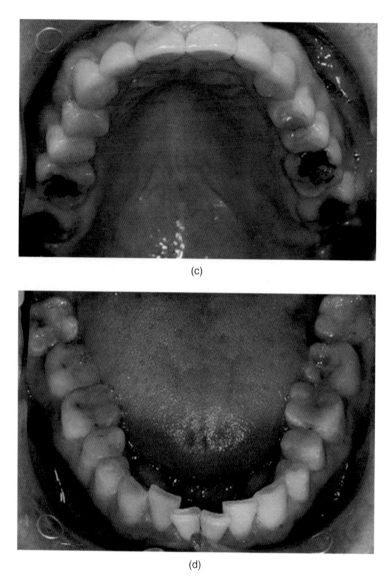

(c)

(d)

Figure 11.3 *(Continued)*

are scalloping of the lateral margins of the tongue and ridging of the buccal cheek mucosa along the occlusal plane. This is due to the soft tissues
being thrust against the surfaces of the teeth during parafunction. Ridging
of the cheek mucosa is occasionally severe enough to present clinically as
frictional hyperkeratosis. Both scalloping of the tongue and ridging of the
cheek mucosa disappear when parafunction ceases, usually within two to
three weeks. In the past, morphological factors such as occlusal discrepancies and the basal bone relationships have been considered principal
aetiological factors for bruxism. More recent control studies have, however, failed to demonstrate any influence of the elimination of occlusal
interferences on bruxist activity.

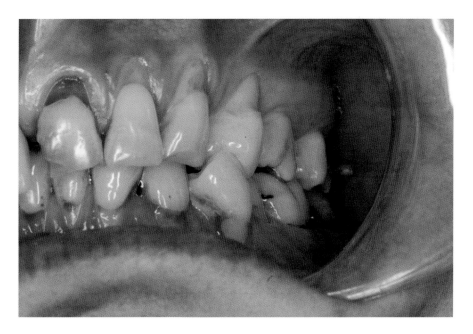

Figure 11.4 Cervical lesions caused by abrasion. (M. Ziad Al-Ani, Robin J.M. Gray.)

Therefore, according to the lack of scientific proof in the role of occlusion on the aetiology of bruxism, this theory has been considered to play only a small role if any. More recent opinion is based on the theory that bruxism appears to be mainly regulated centrally not peripherally. Several studies have demonstrated a high anxiety rate and increased depressive symptoms.

Mild forms of bruxism rarely have any severe consequences for oral structures. In extreme cases, however, bruxism can cause tooth structure breakdown and many authors have suggested that this can play a role in the development of a temporomandibular disorder (TMD).

The most widely accepted management for bruxism is conservative and reversible management including the use of occlusal splints. The soft-tissue signs and general symptoms of bruxism often disappear when occlusal therapy is aimed at careful elimination of interferences in the static and dynamic occlusion and maximal distribution of the occlusal load. The splint of choice is the stabilisation splint. If splint therapy is successful, and the patient is weaned off the appliance, further treatment should be considered only if symptoms return.

Management of attrition

It is important to record the clinical situation. Progression of tooth surface loss can be detected and the effects of preventive measures recorded by a number of methods.

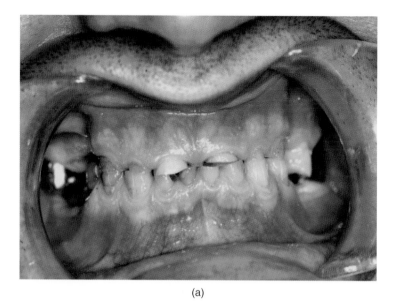

(a)

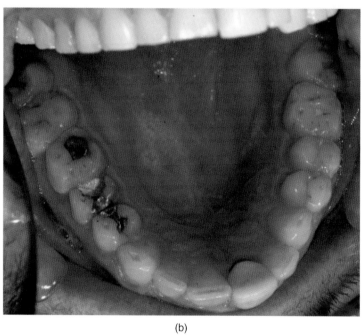

(b)

Figure 11.5 (a) Gross tooth surface loss, (b) toothwear as a result of bruxism showing flattening of cusps, localised facets on occlusal surfaces and fractured restorations. (M. Ziad Al-Ani, Robin J.M. Gray.)

Clinical photographs

These are obviously useful in monitoring wear. Although micro-camera systems are the most versatile and digital intraoral systems are the easiest to use, excellent photographs can be taken with simple equipment.

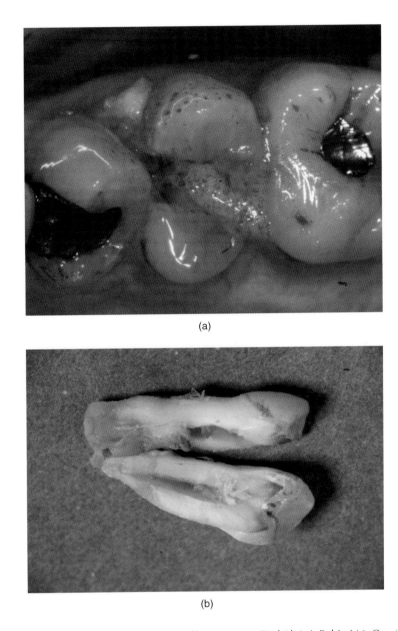

(a)

(b)

Figure 11.6 Tooth fracture as a result of bruxism. (M. Ziad Al-Ani, Robin J.M. Gray.)

Dated reference casts (study models)

These can be used at follow-up visits for comparison with the teeth to monitor wear. Models should be cast with die-stone because they themselves are prone to wear with repeated handling. Due to the potential for discrepancies in impression taking and subsequent casting of the models, precise comparisons cannot be made (Figure 11.7).

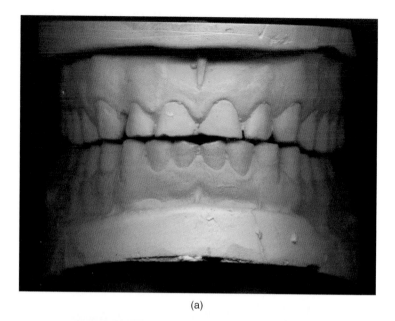

(a)

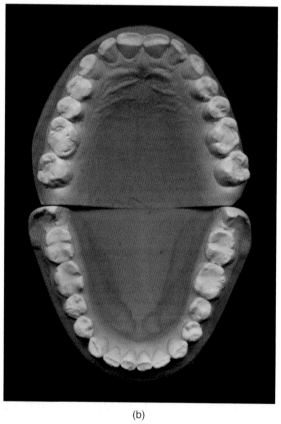

(b)

Figure 11.7 Study models taken for sequential comparison when monitoring tooth surface loss. (M. Ziad Al-Ani, Robin J.M. Gray.)

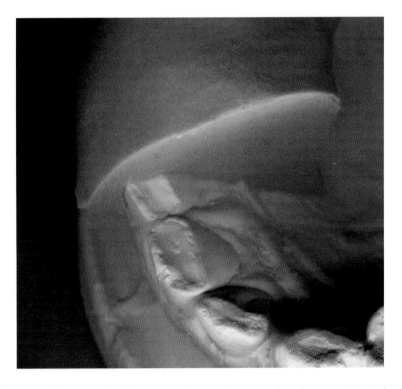

Figure 11.8 The use of a silicone index for monitoring tooth surface loss. (M. Ziad Al-Ani, Robin J.M. Gray.)

Silicone index

A silicone index can be taken of the occlusal surfaces of the teeth. This is dimensionally stable long term and can be placed on subsequent casts or on the patient's teeth for an easy view of potentially worn or wearing sites (Figure 11.8).

Digital 3D scans of teeth obtained over a period of several months or years.

Monitoring can be performed by using a series of digital 3D scans of teeth obtained over a period of several months or years. These digital 3D datasets are also a valuable aid to elucidate the aetiology of the process and explain the nature and severity of the condition to the patients (Figure 11.9).

Determine the cause

It is essential to find the cause of tooth wear. The history taking has to be much more detailed than normal. The following points are especially relevant:

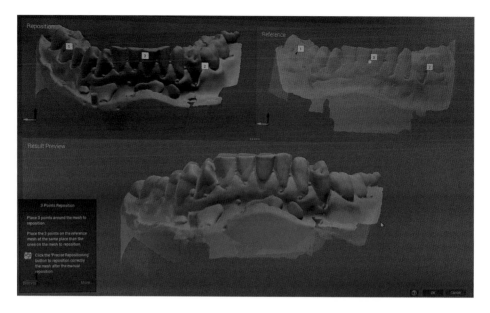

Figure 11.9 The use of digital 3D scans for monitoring tooth surface loss. (M. Ziad Al-Ani, Robin J.M. Gray.)

- Medical history
- Dental hygiene habits
- Lifestyle factors
- History of bruxism.

Prevent and treat the sensitivity

Methods of approaching this include

- Fluoride rinses and mouthwashes
- High-concentration fluoride toothpastes
- Low abrasion toothpaste
- Dentine bonding agents to cover exposed dentine
- Desensitising solutions.

Treatment options

Many treatment options are available and as a general rule, the less good your examination, and the more complex, the treatment plan, the more likely it is to fail. In addition, initial removal of hard tissues such as an occlusal interference should rarely, if ever, be done without a diagnosis and comprehensive treatment plan. Such a procedure does not necessarily lead to a better result.

Categories of tooth surface loss

Category 1

- Appearance satisfactory
- Treatment counselling
- Control of bruxism or clenching habits by means of splint therapy
- Undertake routine restorative care
- Monitor.

Category 2

- Appearance not satisfactory
- No increase in occlusal vertical dimension (OVD) required
- Treatment as for category 1 plus conventional restorative measures, including crowns or composite restorations to deal with aesthetic problems.

Category 3

- Appearance not satisfactory
- Increase in OVD required
- There will be either sufficient or insufficient space available for restorative treatment. This is a very much more complex situation. Vertical tooth height can be lost, but dentoalveolar height may not be lost and the space for restorative treatment may be limited. There is a reduction in the height of the teeth but the lack of space may be due to the compensatory mechanism of dental alveolar compensation. Space therefore needs to be created.

Space for restoration of the occlusion may be obtained in one of three ways:

1. Achieve a generalised increase in OVD by crowning or building up most or all of the teeth in one arch (Figure 11.10).
2. Intrude teeth that require restoration (the Dahl principal).
3. Exploit the difference between centric jaw relation and centric occlusion. In this situation, a record can be made of the first contact in centric jaw relation. Composite can be bonded to the upper and lower anterior teeth to establish occlusal contact in this position. Restoration of the posterior segments can then follow.

Finally, aesthetic restoration of the anterior teeth can be made to this increased vertical dimension. This was the option that the specialist discussed with your patient and along which his treatment progressed.

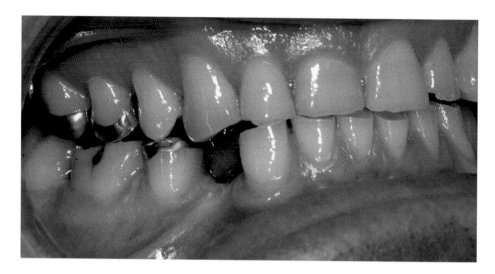

Figure 11.10 Posterior increase of the OVD has been achieved using occlusal gold onlays in a patient with attrition. This will be followed by restoration of anterior segments using an appropriate aesthetic material. (M. Ziad Al-Ani, Robin J.M. Gray.)

A recent proposal for the classification of tooth wear has been introduced by Wetselaar and Lobbezoo. This classification enables the practitioner to distinguish tooth wear based on its distribution (localised or generalised), its severity (mild, moderate, severe, or extreme) and its origin (mechanical/chemical and intrinsic/extrinsic).

Due to the multifactorial nature of the origin of tooth wear, terms like 'mainly' or 'partial' have been added to the origin.

The recent European Consensus Statement on Management Guidelines of severe tooth wear has recommended that "restorative intervention is typically best delayed as long as possible. When such intervention is indicated and agreed upon with the patient, a conservative, minimally invasive approach is recommended, complemented by supportive preventive measures". A protocol to aid decisions on how to best manage patients with severe tooth surface loss has been suggested.

Loss of occlusal vertical dimension, occlusal instability and TMD

Historically, it has been thought that loss of vertical dimension was directly linked to the development of TMD. There is little evidence to support this theory. The most common situation clinically when a gross alteration to vertical dimension can occur is in the complete denture wearer. Patients are often seen who are markedly over-closed, yet this group of patients rarely present with symptoms of a TMD. Similarly, patients who have lost posterior teeth do not have to have them replaced to prevent later development of a TMD. Indeed, the shortened dental arch is often a treatment objective.

Further reading

Bloom, D.R. and Padayachy, J.N. (2006). Increasing occlusal vertical dimension – why, when and how. *Br Dent J* 200: 251–256.

Burke, F.J., Qualtrough, A.J., and Hale, R.W. (1995). The dentine-bonded ceramic crown: an ideal restoration? *Br Dent J* 179: 58–63.

Burke, F.J. (2007). Four year performance of dentine-bonded all ceramic crowns. *Br Dent J* 202: 269–273.

Burke, F.J. (1998). Treatment of loss of tooth substance using dentine-bonded crowns: report of a case. *Dent Update* 25: 235–240.

Davies, S.J., Gray, R.J., and Qualtrough, A.J. (2002). Management of tooth surface loss. *Br Dent J* 192: 11–16. 19–23.

Eccles, J.D. (1982). Tooth surface loss from abrasion, attrition and erosion. *Dent Update* 9: 373–374, 376–8.

Kanno, T. and Carlsson, G.E. (2006). A review of the shortened dental arch concept focusing on the work by the Kayser/Nijmegen group. *J Oral Rehabil* 33: 850–862.

Lerner, J. (2008). A systematic approach to full-mouth reconstruction of the severely worn dentition. *Pract Proced Aesthet Dent* 20: 81–87; quiz 88, 121.

Loomans, B., Opdam, N., Attin, T. et al. (2017). Severe tooth wear: european consensus statement on management guidelines. *J Adhes Dent* 19: 111–119.

Loomans, B. and Opdam, N. (2018). A guide to managing tooth wear: the Radboud philosophy. *Br Dent J* 224: 348–356.

McIntyre, F. (2000). Restoring esthetics and anterior guidance in worn anterior teeth. A conservative multidisciplinary approach. *J Am Dent Assoc* 131: 1279–1283.

Porter, R., Poyser, N., Briggs, P., and Kelleher, M. (2007). Demolition experts: management of the parafunctional patient: 1. Diagnosis and prevention. *Dent Update* 34: 198–200, 202–4, 207.

Poyser, N., Porter, R., Briggs, P., and Kelleher, M. (2007). Demolition experts: management of the parafunctional patient: 2. Restorative management strategies. *Dent Update* 34: 262–264. 266–8.

Poyser, N.J., Porter, R.W., Briggs, P.F. et al. (2005). The Dahl concept: past, present and future. *Br Dent J* 198: 669–676. quiz 720.

Roberts, A. (2008). The use of dentine-bonded crowns in anterior tooth surface loss: a case report. *Dent Update* 35: 622–624. 626.

Robinson, S., Nixon, P.J., Gahan, M.J., and Chan, M.F. (2008). Techniques for restoring worn anterior teeth with direct composite resin. *Dent Update* 35: 551–552. 555–8.

Saha, S. and Summerwill, A.J. (2004). Reviewing the concept of Dahl. *Dent Update* 31: 442–444. 446–7.

Walmsley, D., Walsh, T.F., Lumley, P.J. et al. (2007). *Restorative Dentistry*, 2nde. Churchill, Livingstone: Elsevier.

Wetselaar, P. and Lobbezoo, F. (2016). The tooth wear evaluation system: a modular clinical guideline for the diagnosis and management planning of worn dentitions. *J Oral Rehabil* 43: 69–80.

Chapter 12

I've Got a Headache

Mr Jones, who is a 40-year-old businessman, attends for his routine checkup and examination. He is a regular six-monthly attender and you have known him for several years and have always got on well with him, enjoying chatting about sport, which was a mutual interest.

When he attended on this occasion, however, he appeared distracted and not his normal relaxed self. He explained to you that he had had a throbbing headache off and on for the last couple of months. He had been to his doctor who had prescribed various analgesics but without any lasting benefit. He had read an article in one of the Sunday papers that headache could be associated with tooth grinding and tooth clenching, and he wanted you to examine him and give him your professional opinion as to whether you thought this was possible in his case.

He said that he woke up with a headache every morning and this gradually wore off during the day, only to return later. The painkillers his doctor prescribed were not really helping. He had been under considerable pressure at work because he was worried about redundancy as his company had not been performing very well recently. He said that he had not been sleeping well and on rare occasions he woke in the middle of the night with head pain.

He had been to the optician to have his eyes tested and was told that his prescription had not changed. He had been back to his doctor on several occasions but he felt that his doctor had 'lost interest'. He did remember that he had had a heavy cold recently and he had again been back to his doctor who had prescribed antibiotics because he was concerned that he might have a sinus infection. He had finished two courses of antibiotics but again with no relief of his head pain. His doctor had also checked his ears and found no abnormalities. He had been referred to an ENT consultant who also told Mr Jones that there was nothing wrong with him

Temporomandibular Disorders: A Problem-Based Approach, Second Edition. M. Ziad Al-Ani and Robin J.M. Gray.
© 2021 M. Ziad Al-Ani and Robin J.M. Gray. Published 2021 by John Wiley & Sons Ltd.
Companion Website: www.wiley.com/go/al-ani/temporomandibular-disorders-2e

and that he should have his teeth checked because he might be developing a tooth abscess.

It then became apparent that Mr Jones had two main concerns. The first, and the reason for him being less friendly than usual, was that, as he had been a patient of yours for many years and had been a regular attender, he thought that you might have missed something that had developed to a stage that was now causing him pain and 'if so, you have some explaining to do!'.

He was embarrassed about mentioning his second concern which was that, as no diagnosis had as yet been reached, he was worried that there might be a 'more sinister cause' such as a brain tumour.

Examination

You first examined Mr Jones's teeth and intraoral soft tissues and periodontal condition. His oral hygiene, as usual, was exemplary. He had no calculus and no accumulation of plaque. All soft tissues were healthy in appearance and colour. There was no pocketing and he had a BPE of 1 in all sextants.

While you were examining his dentition, he did volunteer that recently he had had sensitivity of his teeth, not in any specific area but more generalised. He said that this was especially bad when brushing his teeth in the morning and when having his cereal with cold milk, and was one of the factors that led him to believe that he might have a dental problem.

On clinical examination, it was apparent that Mr Jones's mouth was caries free. He only had a few minimal restorations, and there was no evidence of any problems with these. None of his teeth was tender to percussion but he felt that his canines and incisors were generally uncomfortable when you dried them with air from the syringe. There were no obvious wear facets on these teeth. All of his third molar teeth were erupted and in function. There was no evidence of pericoronitis.

Radiographs

You normally only took radiographs of Mr Jones's teeth occasionally in accordance with the IR(ME)R 2018 guidelines. You checked your records and found that you had taken bite-wing radiographs two years previously but, in view of Mr Jones's current concerns, you felt it justifiable to take right and left bite-wing radiographs on this occasion to allay his fears and satisfy yourself that no dental disease had developed.

Bite-wing radiographs were taken which showed there to be no caries and normal bone levels in all four quadrants.

Articulatory system exam 1

You undertook your normal examination of the articulatory system and found him to have discomfort from both right and left temporomandibular joint (TMJ)s on palpation via the external auditory meatus, when he experienced quite sharp discomfort. He also experienced mild discomfort on lateral palpation of the TMJs in the preauricular region on both sides of his face.

His range of vertical mandibular movement was slightly reduced. He could open to 33 mm, but could move his mandible to the right and the left 12 mm in both directions. His pathway of mouth opening was straight, indicating that both joints were acting synchronously.

Having palpated both right and left TMJs and listened to the joints with a stethoscope for joint sounds you could detect neither clicking nor crepitation. You examined the jaw muscles and found mild tenderness of the origin of both right and left masseter muscles along the anterior part of the zygomatic arch, and quite marked tenderness in the anterior fibres of the temporalis muscle.

Even though there was no evidence of clicking at the time of the clinical examination, Mr Jones did say that, for the first time in his life, he had started to get occasional and intermittent jaw joint clicking first thing in the morning. He felt that this was coming mainly from his right TMJ. It did not happen every day and generally disappeared within an hour of waking.

Which muscles are tender?

The jaw muscles are usually tender after parafunction where they insert into bone. The temporalis muscle is frequently found to be tender in patients who grind their teeth, and the masseter muscle is found to be tender in patients who clench their teeth. The posterior belly of the digastric can be tender in those who parafunction on their anterior teeth.

Why do joints click? 4

TMJs exhibit clicking commonly in two clinical situations. First there is a true internal derangement when the intra-articular disc is displaced anteromedially. This gives rise to a consistent click that is always present on opening and closing the mouth and does not come and go.

Second, an intermittent click can be present. If the tonicity of the jaw muscles, especially the superior pterygoid, is increased, it is thought that the intra-articular disc can be pulled forward. This can arise when there is a general increase in muscle activity as seen in patients with parafunctional habits. Increased tone in the superior pterygoid has the effect of displacing the disc forward and medially on a temporary basis.

Most patients who grind or clench their teeth do so at night while asleep and are totally unaware of the habit. After they wake in the morning, there is a decrease in the parafunctional activity, the superior pterygoid gradually relaxes, allowing the elasticity in the posterior bilaminar zone to relocate the disc. The click then disappears and this accounts for the fact that although it is present on waking in the morning it gradually resolves.

Likely diagnosis

In this instance, it is likely that Mr Jones has headaches secondary to a parafunctional habit and associated with a temporomandibular disorder (TMD). Headache is regarded as being a possible TMD symptom but only when accompanied by other signs or symptoms that are indicative of this diagnosis.

Mr Jones presented with headache but also with intermittent TMJ clicking, muscle tenderness, and sensitivity of some of his teeth. This specific group of signs and symptoms would indicate a parafunctional activity possibly caused by the stress that he admitted to being under.

Had he presented with headache as his sole symptom and without any other signs of a TMD or dental disease, then the suggestion you should make would be to refer Mr Jones to a neurologist. This can be done through his general medical practitioner.

Headache

Headache is a symptom. Something causes headache; it is not a disease.

In the Headache Classification Committee of the International Headache Society 2013, the classification and diagnostic criteria for headache disorders, cranial neuralgias, and facial pain give 14 primary headache classifications, each with multiple subdivisions:

- The headache associated with a TMD is listed under classification 2, 'Tension type headache'.
- This is further subdivided into section 2.1: Infrequent episodic tension-type headache
- This is further subdivided into classification 2.1.1: Infrequent episodic tension-type headache associated with pericranial tenderness
- 2.2: Frequent episodic tension-type headache. This is further subdivided into classification 2.2.1 Frequent episodic tension-type headache associated with pericranial tenderness and 2.2.2 Frequent episodic tension-type headache not associated with pericranial tenderness (Figure 12.1).

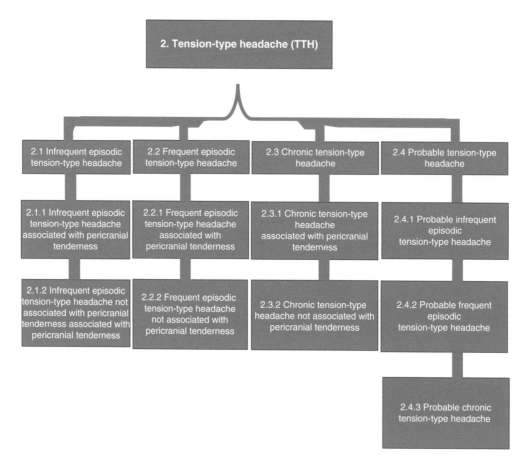

Figure 12.1 Headache classification 2, 'Tension type headache'. (Modified from Headache Classification Committee of the International Headache Society (IHS). The International Classification of Headache Disorders, 3rd edition (beta version). Cephalalgia 2013; 33:629–808.)

This is therefore the *only headache* that dentists are qualified to diagnose and treat. The introduction in *Cephalalgia* makes the following statement:

> The headache of an individual patient may change over a lifetime not only quantitatively but also qualitatively. One patient frequently has more than one form of headache. At one point in a patient's life one form may predominate but later it may be the other. It is a consequence of these problems that it has not been possible to classify patients only to classify headaches' … that we cannot classify patients but only headaches does however introduce other problems. It is not possible to classify all headache episodes in every patient. Most patients have too many, cannot remember them sufficiently well, have taken treatment and so on. Patients always have a number of attacks which cannot be formally classified.

It is therefore the responsibility of the dentist either to diagnose headache associated with a TMD or alternatively eliminate this from a differential diagnosis. If in doubt seek advice!

Dentists should not blindly get involved in the management of patients with headache without having made this judgement. In the absence of these criteria, the correct clinician to treat headache is a neurologist, not a dentist.

As Mr Jones's headache was strongly linked with parafunctional activity with dental sensitivity, intermittent joint clicking, muscle tenderness, and a reduced range of opening, the probable diagnosis is that his headache was associated with either bruxism or clenching. Do not lose sight of the fact that you are treating the TMD not the headache. If the headache also responds so be it, but do not make promises to the patient that you cannot substantiate. Define your treatment objectives clearly in language that the patient understands and make sure that this important point is appreciated.

Management

Do not underestimate the benefit of explanation and reassurance.

Mr Jones attended your surgery thinking that either you had been potentially negligent by allowing a dental problem to develop without treatment or, on a more serious note, he was concerned that none of the clinicians he had seen had been able to put a diagnosis to his problem and there might be a sinister cause, such as a brain tumour. Although this may seem an extreme reaction, it is not unusual in patients who have headache and a TMD, when no diagnosis has been made, to fear the worst. Explain that headache may be a symptom of a TMD or related to parafunction when other TMD symptoms also exist.

Explanation of the problem and the presence of some signs and symptoms such as muscle tenderness and intermittent clicking, tooth sensitivity and scalloping of the buccal mucosa, and ridging of the lateral border of the tongue may elicit a response of 'Now that you mention it, I am aware of grinding or clenching my teeth on occasions but consciously try to stop myself doing it'. Patients frequently report an awareness of parafunctional activity when under stress such as when taking exams, driving, or when in personal or work-related stressful situations.

Drug therapy would not be particularly appropriate.

Mr Jones had been aware of his symptoms only for a short period of time and his principal complaint was headache. He did have some discomfort of some of his jaw muscles and discomfort of his TMJ. What would be more appropriate would be to address the cause of his symptoms rather than merely prescribe drugs to combat the symptoms.

Physiotherapy may be useful in the short term.

He did have some joint and muscle tenderness and decreased opening indicating an inflammatory response in the structures. Physiotherapy in the form of megapulse, acupuncture, or ultrasound could prove beneficial to address the specific symptoms. Excessive exercise or effort should be avoided.

Splint therapy is the best way of approaching management of these symptoms.

There are two types of splints commonly prescribed, either a soft vacuum-formed polyvinyl splint or an occlusally balanced stabilisation splint.

The reason that the soft vacuum-formed splint should be avoided is that, in a number of patients, placing a compressible material between their teeth can actually encourage rather than discourage bruxism or clenching. This appliance is made on the basis that it 'absorbs the force' generated by the jaw muscles. This, however, is not the case. It is thought that by placing a compressible material between the teeth, the force able to be generated actually increases rather than decreases due to the change in proprioception in the periodontal membrane, allowing the individual to generate even more force and subsequently cause more muscle discomfort.

The correct treatment would be to provide a stabilisation splint. To be able to grind the teeth a patient must be able to produce lateral forces against the interdigitated teeth. By providing a stabilisation splint, it is thought that this not only reduces the muscle force generated but also removes the interdigitation between the teeth, allowing the mandible to glide against the splint surface and thereby reduce the impulse to grind the teeth.

It should be explained to the patient that this design of appliance has a success rate in the region of 80–85% but unfortunately it is impossible to predict the 10–15% or so in whom they do not work. Once fitted and correctly balanced, such an appliance can be kept long term and used on an 'as-needed' basis.

Patient journey

Mr Jones presented with a distressing and, he felt, potentially serious complaint. He was also concerned that his dentist had possibly been negligent because of the advice that he had been given by a third party (the ENT consultant).

After careful history taking, examination, and explanation and reassurance, Mr Jones was comfortable with the fact that his headache was secondary to a parafunctional activity and associated with a TMD.

A stabilisation splint was made, fitted, and balanced, and his symptoms resolved.

Due to the ongoing nature of the stressful situation that he was in, he could use this splint on an as-needed basis and he was comfortable and reassured by the outcome of the treatment plan.

Further Reading

Gray, R.J., Davies, S.J., and Quayle, A.A. (1994). A clinical approach to temporomandibular disorders. 8. Should dentists treat headache? *Br Dent J* 177: 255–259.

Headache Classification Committee of the International Headache Society (IHS) (2013). The international classification of headache disorders, 3rd edition (beta version). *Cephalalgia* 33: 629–808.

The Ionising Radiation (Medical Exposure) Regulations 2018. Available at: https://www.legislation.gov.uk/uksi/2018/121/introduction/made

Olesen, J. and Steiner, T.J. (2004). The international classification of headache disorders, 2nd edn (ICDH-II). *J Neurol Neurosurg Psychiatry* 75: 808–811.

Chapter 13

I've Got Whiplash

One of your patients, Diane Green, attends your surgery one morning. She has been booked in as an emergency patient because she has recently broken a tooth that is very sensitive not only to bite on but also to temperature. She has been a patient of yours for many years and, although she has had no clinical treatment completed recently, she does have a heavily restored dentition.

When you examined her you found that the palatal cusp of the upper right first molar had fractured sublingually and was being retained in place only by the gingival tissues. The tooth itself was not tender to percussion but it was very sensitive to move the mobile fractured palatal cusp. In addition, the tooth exhibited hypersensitivity when you blew cold air on it.

She sat in the chair but requested to be treated upright because she had recently been involved in a road traffic accident (RTA) and her back, shoulders, and neck were very stiff. She thinks it was in this accident that she broke the tooth.

As the appointment was only relatively short your initial clinical treatment plan was to give her a palatal injection of local anaesthetic, remove the mobile fractured cusp and place a temporary dressing over the exposed dentine. You did discuss with her that a full coverage crown would probably be necessary, but that the treatment that you were about to undertake would give her relief from her symptoms both of discomfort when she bit down on the tooth and of thermal sensitivity. She was quite happy with this treatment plan but, when you asked her to open as wide as she could, so you were able to administer a palatal injection, she said that her jaw was very stiff and would open only about one and a half fingers' width. On questioning her she said that there was pain in her jaw joint on the left side but also that she felt that her jaw 'would not go' as

Temporomandibular Disorders: A Problem-Based Approach, Second Edition. M. Ziad Al-Ani and Robin J.M. Gray.
© 2021 M. Ziad Al-Ani and Robin J.M. Gray. Published 2021 by John Wiley & Sons Ltd.
Companion Website: www.wiley.com/go/al-ani/temporomandibular-disorders-2e

there was a physical obstruction to her opening wide. She did volunteer that her jaw had been like this since the time of the accident. She also said that she had had to go on to soft diet because chewing was painful, not just as a result of the fractured upper molar tooth. She said that it was also difficult to yawn.

When you asked her about the accident, she told you that she was the driver of her own car and she was wearing a seatbelt. She was not aware of striking her head anywhere on the inside of the car but she was hit in a rear-end shunt when she stopped at a roundabout to let traffic pass. She said the impact was severe enough to render her car (the target vehicle) and the other car (the bullet vehicle) impossible to drive. She was aware of her head being 'whipped back' to hit the headrest, propelled forward against the seatbelt restraint and then her head forcibly snapping back again to strike the head restraint. She remembers her mouth closing with a sudden severe force and she feels that this is what was responsible for the fractured molar. The accident happened about a week before you saw her. Initially she had gone to her GP because her neck and shoulders were very 'tense' and he prescribed a non-steroidal anti-inflammatory agent (ibuprofen). It was two to three days later, when her neck symptoms began to plateau and improve slightly, that she became aware of the problems with her jaw.

Examination 1

Once you had resolved her immediate dental problem, which was difficult for you both because of poor access, you examined the rest of the articulatory system and found that there was a very occasional click from her left temporomandibular joint (TMJ). She was able to open slightly wider after the click but mostly she was only able to open to about 17 mm. When she opened and experienced locking, she showed an obvious lasting deviation to the left side. When her jaw locked she did not click. The click was audible only with the use of a stethoscope. There was tenderness of her jaw muscles (masseter, lateral pterygoid, and temporalis). There was only mild tenderness on lateral palpation of the TMJs but there was acute tenderness on intra-auricular palpation of the left TMJ via the external auditory meatus. You confined yourself to examination of her jaw muscles because you felt that examination of the muscles of the cervical spine and the shoulder girdle was outwith your area of expertise.

You tried to examine her occlusion, but, due to her inability to comfortably move her mandible, you felt that the results of a comprehensive occlusal examination would be unreliable. From previous examinations, there were no obvious factors of note that you felt could be contributing to her symptoms. She had no signs of bruxism in that there was no ridging of the buccal mucosa, scalloping of the edge of the tongue or marked attrition, and she was not aware of any habit.

Radiographic examination

You did not feel that an intraoral radiograph would be of any benefit and you had in fact taken bite-wing radiographs six months previously.

Record-keeping

You felt that accurate record-keeping would be mandatory in this situation. You have always been very careful keeping records but you are aware of the fact, from your conversation, that a legal case was pending in view of her accident and you realised that at some, possibly much later stage, you would be required to produce accurate and contemporaneous notes. It was important therefore to record all factors relevant to the articulatory system, in addition to the damage to her teeth and the timescale of the onset of her symptoms in relation to the RTA.

One final feature to note is that, if a cervical spine injury has been severe, the person may attribute all the symptoms in the face and neck to the neck injury and become aware of the presence of temporomandibular disorder (TMD) symptoms only as other symptoms from the cervical spine start to improve; the patient might not be aware of them initially. You may therefore only hear about development of these symptoms some time later.

It has been suggested that as many as one of four patients with TMD has a history of head/neck trauma in proximity to the development of their TMD pain

The term whiplash expresses the characteristic head and neck motion that occurs when a relatively rigid thorax is suddenly accelerated or decelerated independently of the head. It simply describes a hyper-extension/flexion injury to the soft tissues of the neck. It would suggest that after the hyper-extension phase, a rebound or recoil injury in hyper-flexion occurs, hence the use of the term 'whiplash'. The typical situation in which this can occur is when the occupant of a motor vehicle undergoes a sudden collision, typically in an RTA when the front end of one car (the bullet vehicle) strikes the rear end of another car (target vehicle). It is believed that the injury is not the result of direct physical impact forces or direct trauma to the occupant of the vehicle by contact with an object inside the target vehicle; rather it is suggested as being an indirect physical reaction to forward acceleration of the target vehicle, namely indirect trauma, released through acceleration/deceleration of the occupant's head, neck, and mandible. The result may be bony or soft tissue injuries or both and this may lead to a variety of clinical manifestations which are grouped under the name 'whiplash associated disorder'.

Unfortunately, these disorders are poorly defined. The signs include a wide range of often semi-covert injuries but symptoms vary widely. Many injuries cannot be detected by radiographic or even manual examination. It has been postulated that the severity of the whiplash associated disorder may be affected by many factors such as vehicle type, restraint type, seatbelts or lap straps, airbags and headrests, the occupant's position in the vehicle, the type, the angle, and the speed of impact, and the degree of structural damage.

It has also been suggested that a degree of damage can be related to whether or not the accident victim had the time to brace themselves if they could see the impact coming and whether or not they had their mouth open at the time of impact.

Are TMD and whiplash related?

This is a highly controversial topic and one on which the literature is not clear. Generally, there are a limited number of studies reporting on the prevalence of TMD related to neck trauma, and thus, there is currently a gap in the knowledge in this area.

A recent systematic review suggested that the prevalence of whiplash trauma is higher in patients with TMD compared with controls, and TMD patients with comorbid TMD/whiplash have more jaw pain and more severe jaw dysfunction, compared with TMD patients without a history of neck injury. The authors concluded that whiplash trauma might be an initiating and/or aggravating factor as well as a comorbid condition for TMD.

There are several factors to consider, the principal ones being traumatic, physiological, psychological, and cultural.

Trauma

When considering the trauma to the articulatory system in an RTA/whiplash injury, there are two types of trauma that must be considered: direct trauma and indirect trauma. Some believe that, without evidence of direct trauma to the face and jaws, subsequent development of a TMD cannot be related to the accident. Others, however, believe that indirect trauma can result after acceleration and deceleration of the person's head, neck, and mandible. This can produce soft-tissue injuries that are not detectable by radiograph and can cause clinical symptoms.

Physiological

If there is direct trauma to the mandible, a traumatic arthritis can arise within the joint which can cause an intracapsular inflammatory exudate, with subsequent pain and restricted movement. If there is sudden stretching of the muscles, muscle pain and spasm can result

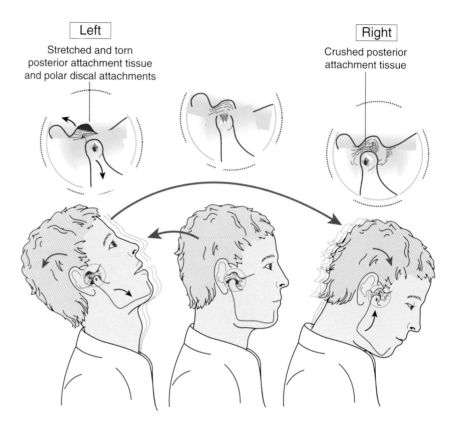

Figure 13.1 Perceived head and neck movement following whiplash. (Weinberg S, Lapointe H. Cervical extension–flexion injury (whiplash) and internal derangement of the temporomandibular joint. J Oral Maxillofac Surg 1987;45:653–6 © ,1987 Elsevier.)

and, as the intra-articular disc is attached to the superior pterygoid, disc displacement can result.

In the case of indirect trauma, it is thought that, as the head and cervical spine are forced back in the hyperextension phase of the injury, the mandible lags behind, thus putting considerable strain on the musculature, capsule, and capsular attachments and resulting in soft-tissue injury. The second phase of this indirect trauma is thought to be during hyperflexion when the head and cervical spine move rapidly forward so that the mandible closes forcibly. This can itself cause direct compression on the disc and result in dental trauma such as Mrs Green experienced when the upper and lower teeth closed forcibly (Figure 13.1).

It has been suggested that development of an internal derangement after a whiplash injury is as a direct result of trauma to the mandible in that the pull of the lateral pterygoid muscle in combination with the force of the trauma causes stretching of the posterior attachment of the disc and a resultant antro-medial displacement. It is thought that this is particularly significant if the trauma occurred when the mouth was open. The literature, however, is at variance in relation to cause and effect.

Psychological

It has been reported that some patients develop a 'late-onset' TMD after an acute whiplash hyperextension/hyperflexion injury and that this is psychosomatic; a degree of symptom amplification has occurred as the person enters a chronic phase after an acute injury.

It has been suggested that therapists need to be compassionate and recognise the validity of the symptoms and that there may be various physical causes. They should be able to advise that various chronic symptoms can arise from a patient's response to the initial problem.

Cultural

There are considerable cultural differences in relation to claims for damages and treatment costs in relation to whiplash injury. This is especially so in relation to development of late-onset TMD. Not surprisingly, those who live in societies where litigation is commonplace are more likely to seek advice, treatment, and subsequent legal redress.

Likely diagnosis

You had known Mrs Green for many as her dentist. She had seen you every six months. You had never recorded any signs or symptoms of a TMD, even though you routinely examined her articulatory system.

She had never experienced reduction in mouth opening, discomfort from her TMJs or masticatory muscles, or TMJ clicking. It is therefore likely, on the balance of probabilities, that her current TMD symptoms arose as a direct result of the RTA.

Management

Mrs Green's clinical management is the same for any other patient with an acute TMD that may have a traumatic origin.

She appears to have an unstable disc within the TMJ, in that on most occasions she has TMJ locking whereas on some occasions she has TMJ clicking. Sometimes her mouth opening is markedly restricted and at other times it is less so. The disc would therefore appear to be unstable. She has muscle tenderness. Her initial management should be explanation, reassurance and immediate referral for outpatient physiotherapy to address the inflammation of the joints and the pain from the muscles.

Splint therapy would not be appropriate at this stage in her management. Provision of a soft polyvinyl vacuum form splint may increase muscle discomfort. An anterior repositioning splint should be avoided in the acute phase when the disc is obviously unstable. Provision of an occlusally balanced stabilisation splint would not be possible if the disc were not in position.

Drug therapy

Temazepam 10 mg at night, half an hour before going to sleep, is a useful muscle relaxant in somebody who has acute pterygoid spasm. This dose must not be exceeded. The drug should be prescribed with the doctor's knowledge and agreement for 10–14 days using a lesser dose if possible while still being therapeutic. Therapy should be discontinued sooner if symptoms resolve. Benzodiazepines have a recognised pharmacological muscle relaxant effect. This may help to allow the disc to reposition by lessening the pull from the superior pterygoid.

Ibuprofen 400 mg three times a day can be prescribed as an anti-inflammatory agent. Patients should be counselled that they must take this regularly after food for two to three days before the anti-inflammatory effect will be realised. If it is taken on an 'as-needed' basis, it is no more effective than paracetamol.

Physiotherapy

Immediate referral to a physiotherapist will provide Mrs Green with the most relief. An exercise programme should be avoided during the acute phase of the condition due to the instability of the disc because the risk of exacerbating the disc displacement is significant. Megapulse, ultrasound, soft laser and acupuncture are all commonly employed therapies. For treatment to be most successful appointments should be arranged two to three times a week for two to three weeks, totalling 8–10 sessions in all. The choice of which particular modality is to be used is up to the physiotherapist. Mrs Green should be monitored at regular intervals to ensure that her symptoms resolve. You should remember that, as the stage and symptoms of the disorder vary, the treatment plan may need to be varied alongside the current situation.

Although splint therapy is not appropriate at the onset it may be a valuable treatment at a later stage.

Notes on management of patients present with clinical signs and symptoms of a temporomandibular disorder following a whiplash injury

- the disorder should be treated as one would treat any other similar TMD, noting the potential trauma from the whiplash injury
- The date, time and circumstances of the accident should be noted as well as the date of onset of symptoms.

- keep strict records of the onset of the symptoms in relation to the date and time of the initial injury and keep accurate follow up records. Notes should also be made of effect of the symptoms on day to day function such as diet, chewing and yawning, the effect on hobbies and other quality of life aspects and any perceived disruption to the occlusion.
- Due to the force of the impact, patients may present with broken teeth or broken restorations. This occurs because during the hyperextension phase of the injury, the mandible 'lags behind' the rest of the skull and during of the hyper flexion phase, the mandible forcibly closes causing an impact between the upper and lower teeth. In these circumstances direct trauma to the dental tissues is not unusual and should be noted.
- The patient may become aware of acute symptoms immediately after the time of the accident. This will normally be manifest by inability to open the mouth comfortably, inability to chew, forced change to a soft diet and pain from the areas of the mandibular muscles or from the joints themselves.
- It is also not uncommon for a click to develop immediately after a whiplash injury due to severe symptoms from the cervical spine, the TMD symptoms might not become apparent until the pain from other structures subsides. This can take three to four weeks from the time of the accident.
- Symptoms may well have been present since the time of the impact but have been masked by the severity of the other problems.

Further Reading

Boniver, R. (2002). Temporomandibular joint dysfunction in whiplash injuries: association with tinnitus and vertigo. *Int Tinnitus J* 8: 129–131.

Gola, R., Richard, O., Guyot, L., and Cheynet, F. (2004). Whiplash lesions and temporomandibular joint disorders. *Rev Stomatol Chir Maxillofac* 105: 274–282.

Sale, H. and Isberg, A. (2007). Delayed temporomandibular joint pain and dysfunction induced by whiplash trauma: a controlled prospective study. *J Am Dent Assoc* 138: 1084–1091.

Weinberg, S. and Lapointe, H. (1987). Cervical extension–flexion injury (whiplash) and internal derangement of the temporomandibular joint. *J Oral Maxillofac Surg* 45: 653–656.

Evidence-based Dentistry

Haggman -Henrikson, B., Rezvani, M., and List, T. (2014). Prevalence of whiplash trauma in TMD patients: a systematic review. *J Oral Rehabil* 41: 59–68.

Chapter 14

What's of Use to Me in Practice?

When considering management of any patient with a temporomandibular disorder (TMD), it is pointless trying to evolve a treatment plan that is either impractical, on the one hand, or unnecessary, on the other.

You are the patient's general dental practitioner and in most instances you will have known the patient for some period of time. You will therefore be aware of treatment needs and expectations more accurately than the specialist whom the patient is seeing for the first time. It is pointless prescribing an anterior repositioning splint for a young patient that, to be successful, must be worn 24 hours a day if you know that the patient won't comply with the usage instructions. Similarly, if you do refer your patient on for a specialist opinion, if appropriate, ask for a practice-based treatment plan if you wish to undertake the management yourself and it is within the remit of your experience. Alternatively, refer for an opinion and treatment. Always monitor what is being done for your patient elsewhere and be aware of the treatment objectives and proposed outcome.

In the vast majority of patients with TMD, the prognosis is favourable. Long-term follow-up of patients with TMD shows that 75–85% of the patients with chronic pain are cured or improve significantly irrespective of the treatment modality used.

It is important to develop a tailored treatment protocol aiming to manage pain and function.

A combination of treatments may often be employed. There appear to be synergistic effects with, for example, a combination of splint therapy, outpatient physiotherapy, and muscle relaxant pharmacotherapy often producing a better result than any of the individual options used in isolation.

Temporomandibular Disorders: A Problem-Based Approach, Second Edition. M. Ziad Al-Ani and Robin J.M. Gray.
© 2021 M. Ziad Al-Ani and Robin J.M. Gray. Published 2021 by John Wiley & Sons Ltd.
Companion Website: www.wiley.com/go/al-ani/temporomandibular-disorders-2e

Counselling and reassurance

This demands a sympathetic clinician, an understandable explanation of the problem and its possible multifactorial aetiology, and a carefully explained and justified course of action, if only to dispel the common fears such as cancer, or that surgery is necessarily the only way forward.

Never underestimate the importance of this. Your patient should have his or her symptoms explained in simple terms that he or she can understand. The treatment objectives should equally be explained and the fact that you may change the treatment plan part way through your management, in response to how the patient's symptoms alter as time passes.

Discussing parafunctional activity is also important for raising a patient's awareness and may improve their condition and consequently able to control it.

Drug therapy

The two groups of drugs normally employed in the management of patients with TMDs are benzodiazepines and non-steroidal anti-inflammatory drugs (NSAIDs). Benzodiazepines have a useful muscle relaxant effect and it is preferable to prescribe them in liquid form, such as Temazepam Oral Suspension, so that patients can titrate their own dose and feel the benefits of the muscle relaxation without any 'hangover' (see Chapter 6). A prescription should be given with the knowledge of the patient's GP and the patient should be counselled that benzodiazepines are licensed as anxiolytics, not as muscle relaxants, although they do have a recognised pharmacological muscle relaxant effect. They are not licensed for prescription to patients aged under 12 years.

Most patients will have already self-prescribed NSAIDs such as ibuprofen or will have been advised to take these.

Generally, NSAIDs have limited success. Ibuprofen is a mild NSAID, but has only mild side effects. It can be useful in the management of chronic pain but its use is limited and, if taken on an 'as needed' basis, is no better than paracetamol.

When prescribing NSAIDs, they should be taken regularly three times a day after food. It will be some days before the maximum anti-inflammatory effect is realised.

The usual prescription is Ibuprofen, 400 mg three times per day for up to one month. Patients should be counselled that it may take from 3 to 5 days before the anti-inflammatory effect is realised.

NSAIDs must not be prescribed to any patient with a history of asthma or gastric irritation including peptic ulceration. Prescription of these drugs without checking the medical history is negligent.

Paracetamol prescribed in a stepwise manner alongside NSAIDs may help reduce the need for NSAIDs and therefore limit their side effects.

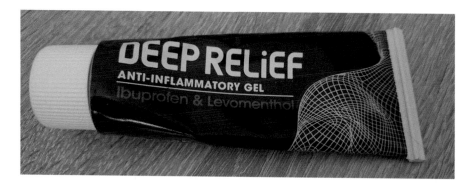

Figure 14.1 Anti-inflammatory gel containing Ibuprofen and Levomenthol. (M. Ziad Al-Ani, Robin J.M. Gray.)

Anti-inflammatory gel (preferably containing Ibuprofen and Levomenthol) can be used in some cases (Figure 14.1). When a patient has localised areas of muscle or joint tenderness, this gel can be massaged into the skin over the affected area. It contains Ibuprofen as an anti-inflammatory agent (stimulates blood flow) and Levomenthol which can trigger the cold-sensitive receptors giving a cooling sensation to the affected area.

 Tricyclic antidepressant drugs cannot be prescribed by general dental practitioners and should be used with caution in the management of TMDs.

If a patient presents with a specific area of acute muscle spasm, which is readily identifiable by digital palpation, a vapo-coolant spray, such as ethyl chloride can be used for temporary relief (Figure 14.2). This should be administered in the surgery environment.

Ethyl chloride spray is applied to the painful areas for approximately five seconds.

The muscle is then gently stretched and this can be used for temporary relief from acute muscle spasm. The eyes, nose, and ears are protected from the spray.

The available literature suggest that there is insufficient evidence to support or not support the effectiveness of the reported drugs for the management of pain due to TMD. Sufficient data do not exist upon which pharmacological intervention can be based. In the interim, dentists who treat TMD patients should consider the use of many drug classes as being 'non-validated' clinical practice. Considerable difference of opinion exists about the efficacy of different drugs and clinicians, therefore, are at present unable to make informed treatment decisions that will effectively manage pain.

Physiotherapy

 As with any musculoskeletal injury, physiotherapy has a large part to play in the patient's successful management.

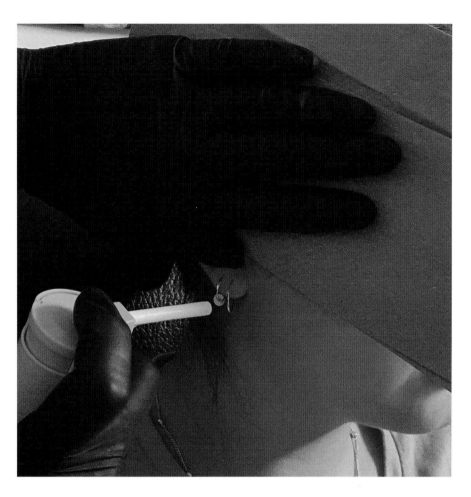

Figure 14.2 Ethyl chloride spray is applied to the painful area. The eyes, nose, and ears should be protected from the spray. (M. Ziad Al-Ani, Robin J.M. Gray.)

The available literature suggests that physiotherapy started early in the course of any musculo-skeletal disorder significantly reduces the duration of symptoms.

This treatment option is beneficial to any TMD patient when there is muscle involvement.

If a patient presents with an acute TMD, immediate referral for physiotherapy should be considered. Leave the choice of the physiotherapy treatment up to the therapist, but suggest that during the acute phase of the disorder excessive exercise should be avoided if there is a question of disc displacement. The usually employed modalities of outpatient electro-physiotherapy are megapulse and ultrasound. Soft laser is also used.

Recent research suggests that either manual therapy or electrical modality intervention would be an option for the treatment of TMD to improve functional outcomes.

The course must be intensive. The ideal frequency of appointments is two to three times a week for three to four weeks, totalling 8–10 sessions in all, but leave this to the discretion of the physiotherapist. Once a week will have much less benefit.

The patient should be advised to treat the TMD as if they had sprained any other joint and rest should be suggested rather than aggressive attempts to increase the range of movement. To do so could compromise the integrity of the intra-articular disc, depending on the particular diagnosis.

Aggressive exercise during an acute TMD phase is best avoided owing to the potential for possible further damage to a displaced disc or inflamed muscle. If the acute symptoms have resolved and there is a residual deviation or restriction on opening, closing, or on protrusion, then remedial exercises can be advised to correct the deviation. These should be done in the vertical, lateral, and antero-posterior directions. The patient should stand in front of a mirror, place one hand over the side of the mandible towards which the deviation is occurring and then open, close, or protrude the lower jaw, applying hand pressure to ensure the mandible moves in a straight line. These are all useful 'corrective' exercises. During the acute phase, however, a patient should be told to treat his/her TMD as similar to a sprain and should rest the mandible as much as possible, keep to a soft diet, and avoid vigorous exercise.

Splint therapy 7

 The soft lower vacuum formed splint is commonly used but cannot be made to any prescription. Usually, an impression of the opposing arch is not even made. It is suggested that these appliances either have a placebo effect or in some way 'absorb' the forces generated by the muscles. What does tend to happen in practice is that these appliances increase parafunction in a number of patients, thereby making the clinical symptoms worse. It is not unusual for a patient to return for review, having bitten completely through the surface of such an appliance (Figure 14.3).

 The anterior repositioning splint is a useful appliance for patients who have a click from the temporomandibular joint (TMJ) that disappears on protrusion of the mandible. This appliance needs to be worn 24 hours a day, to be removed only for cleaning after eating and should be used for approximately 12 weeks. A gradual weaning-off process should be used (Figure 14.4).

The patient should stop wearing the appliance if the jaw locks or if any part breaks off because this latter situation could allow tooth movement.

 The localised occlusal interference splint can be used for patients who grind or clench their teeth but only for those who do so in centric occlusion. If a patient performs parafunction at extreme lateral movements, this appliance will immediately be rendered inactive because it will not contact during the parafunctional activity (Figure 14.5).

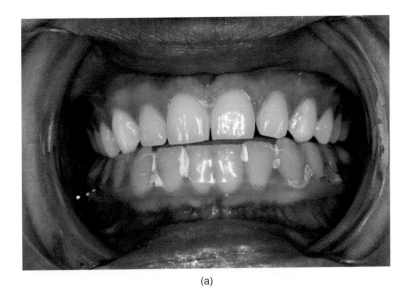

(a)

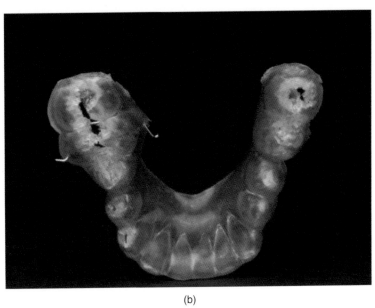

(b)

Figure 14.3 Soft bite guard after being worn by someone with bruxism for 3 months. (From Gray RJ, Davies SJ. Emergency treatment of acute temporomandibular disorders: Part I. Dent Update 1997;24:170–3, with permission).

 The stabilisation splint is the definitive splint for those with occlusal discrepancies or marked parafunctional activity. Ideally, it is constructed to eliminate posterior occlusal interferences, provide anterior guidance on anterior teeth, and provide contacts when centric relation and centric occlusion coincide. This is a successful appliance for patients who have a parafunctional input to their symptoms. It needs to be worn only at night and after the initial period of usage can be gradually discontinued until it is used only on an as-needed basis (Figure 14.6).

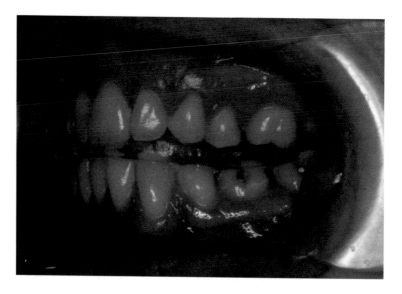

Figure 14.4 Anterior repositioning splint in place with incisors in edge-to-edge relationship. (Note the full coverage of all occlusal surfaces.) (M. Ziad Al-Ani, Robin J.M. Gray.)

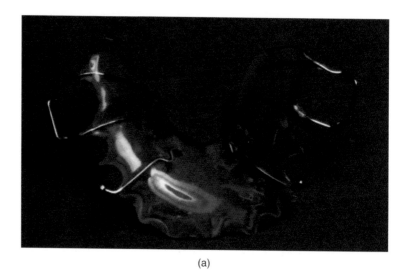

(a)

Figure 14.5 Localised occlusal interference splint for patients who clench or parafunction in centric occlusion. (M. Ziad Al-Ani, Robin J.M. Gray.)

 There is no place in the management of patients with TMD for a partial coverage appliance because this can allow unpredictable tooth movement. Such appliances are medicolegally indefensible.

One exception to this rule is when a Dhal appliance is involved as part of a patient's treatment to encourage controlled and predetermined tooth movement as part of an overall treatment plan.

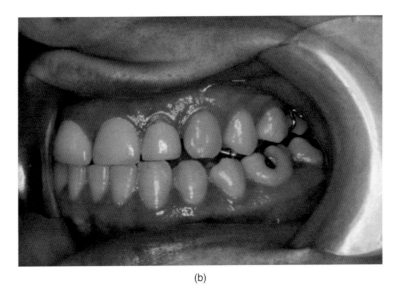

(b)

Figure 14.5 *(Continued)*

Mouth prop

The use of a mouth prop is very helpful for patients who have a TMD irrespective of the diagnosis. The benefit of a mouth prop during extended periods of dental treatment, or even visits to the dental hygienist, should not be underestimated. This is not just because it is more comfortable for the patient but because, by employing our knowledge of anatomy, we can appreciate the rationale behind its use. If a susceptible patient is asked to open and/or protrude the mouth over a period of time without the use of a mouth prop, the lateral pterygoid muscle contracts. This can predispose to anterior displacement of the intra-articular disc. If, however, the patient is asked to rest against a mouth prop, the elevator muscles of the mandible become active with the lateral pterygoid muscles, among others, being less so (Figure 14.7).

Occlusal adjustments

Occlusal adjustments may be tempting. If there is obvious interference, in the past it has been suggested that 'picking up a hand piece and removing the interference' may lead to an improvement in the patient's symptoms. This, however, is a dangerous course of action if previous analysis of mounted study casts and a plaster equilibration has not been undertaken. Otherwise, removal of premature contacts or interferences will be merely guesswork. It is similar to the analogy of sawing the legs off a table without any measurement. If part is removed from one leg it is frequently necessary to form repeated adjustments to the other three legs until a stable position is reached, if indeed it can be.

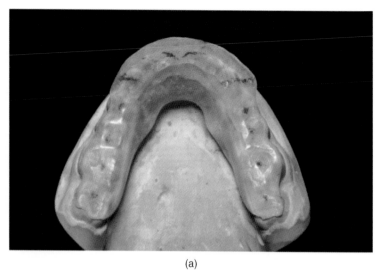

(a)

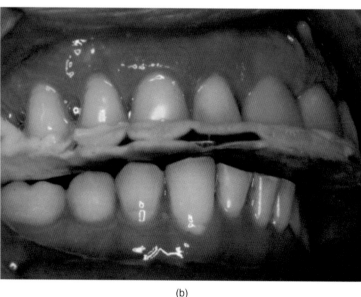

(b)

Figure 14.6 (a) Lower stabilisation splint balanced to centric relation/occlusion. (b) Upper stabilisation splint in place. (M. Ziad Al-Ani, Robin J.M. Gray.)

 Medicolegally, it is difficult to defend haphazard removal of tooth substance or the surface of crowns or other restorations in an attempt to alter the occlusion, if this has not been pre-planned, and it should therefore be avoided. Caution should be adopted in the use of occlusal adjustment as a remedy for TMD as this can cause medico-legal concerns.

It is apparent when treating a patient with an occlusally balanced appliance that the mandibular position can alter quite markedly as treatment progresses and painful muscles relax. For this reason, what initially might be deemed to be an occlusal interference or premature contact at the onset

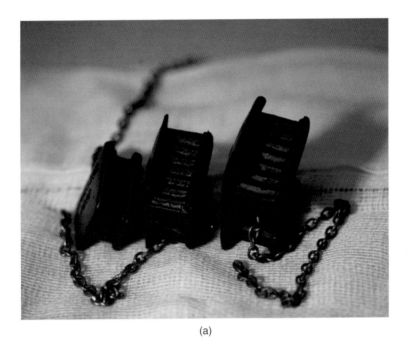

(a)

(b)

Figure 14.7 Mouth prop for use in patient with temporomandibular disorder when having dental treatment. (M. Ziad Al-Ani, Robin J.M. Gray.)

of treatment might not be one at the end. As an initial therapy, occlusal adjustment is therefore not recommended as jaw and tooth relationships cannot be accurately determined in the presence of pain. The approach of 'pick up a handpiece and remove interferences at the first visit' is not defensible. It would therefore appear to be sound advice not to make permanent and irreversible adjustment to the occlusion in the presence of a TMD as when the disc is repositioned occlusal contacts will change.

There is insufficient evidence to suggest that any occlusal treatment is as, or more effective than any other rehabilitation treatment in TMD. There is also insufficient evidence to support the generalised preventive influence of occlusal adjustment or orthodontic correction of malocclusion on TMD development.

Evidence based studies showed that there was an absence of evidence from RCTs that occlusal adjustments prevent or treat a TMD and, therefore, occlusal adjustment cannot be recommended for the management or prevention of TMD and future trials should use standardised diagnostic criteria and outcome measures when evaluating TMD.

In general, the literature suggests that occlusal equilibration, therefore, should not be provided as an initial therapy for TMD patients and occlusal equilibration should not be performed to prevent or treat signs or symptoms.

It has also been suggested that if an anterior repositioning appliance successfully treats symptoms of an internal derangement then the occlusion should be restored to the treatment position. Contrary to what some practitioners advocate, however, occlusal therapy is not needed to maintain a TMD patient's long-term symptomatic improvement.

Since occlusal treatments are typically irreversible and the evidence on their therapeutic or preventive effects on TMD is insufficient, it is recommended that reversible treatment such as self-care, splints, physiotherapy, and pharmacotherapy should always be used initially to manage signs and symptoms of TMD. As symptoms of pain and dysfunction in a TMD patient may come and go without any obvious change in any recognisable factor, one must be very hesitant about introducing any permanent changes in any part of the system.

Irreversible occlusal adjustment should never be undertaken in the presence of acute muscle pain or TMD symptoms. Ideally, occlusal adjustments should not be done until after a period of successful splint treatment. If a well-balanced stabilisation splint is worn and the patient's symptoms resolve, only to return when the splint is 'weaned off', then there might be a logical reason to address the occlusion of the natural teeth, but not without further and detailed occlusal analysis and only after meticulous planning with articulated plaster casts and with informed consent. This would indicate whether provision of an 'improved' occlusion would benefit the patient's symptoms.

If occlusal adjustment or equilibration is deemed necessary for other clinical reasons then this should always be planned on study models mounted on a semi-adjustable articulator before irreversible and permanent changes are made to the patient's natural dentition.

In this way, the sequence of alterations can be carefully planned, and it can also be determined whether the desired result is actually achievable.

It is acknowledged that occlusal treatment can be used successfully to correct an uncomfortable occlusion in a patient with or without TMD. For example, a patient who reports an uncomfortably high, recently placed restoration can be treated with occlusal adjustment of this restoration as the primary treatment.

Given that there are other, less invasive approaches available, and TMD symptoms may be self-limiting, it would seem that occlusal adjustment is not indicated unless additional evidence is forthcoming.

When planning alterations to a patient's occlusion, either a conformative or reorganised approach can be undertaken. This is a large subject and is outwith the remit of this text. It should be noted, however, that iatrogenic introduction of occlusal interferences can lead to the development of a TMD. Occlusal rehabilitation is not a treatment need for all patients, as patients can function perfectly well with missing functional units.

Remember that it is often a combination of the above treatments that will suit your patient's individual needs best, so you must remain adaptable and gear your plan to the current state of the disorder. Some treatments that may have previously been therapeutic may become detrimental if the clinical presentation alters.

Does orthodontic treatment cause TMD? 12

Currently, and based on the available evidence, the role of orthodontic treatment in the aetiology of TMD is not confirmed. The hypothesis that different orthodontic techniques and treatment plans can be involved as aetiological factors for TMD has also been tested in recent decades. Neither orthodontic treatment nor extraction showed a causal relationship with the signs and symptoms of TMD.

The orthodontist has been both accused of causing, and complimented for curing, a TMD. The available literature indicates that a significant percentage of professional negligence actions against orthodontists include allegations of failure to diagnose a TMD, failure to provide timely treatment or failure to refer.

Orthodontists are advised to develop and to implement a specific protocol for the management of patients who develop signs or symptoms of a TMD either before, during, or after orthodontic treatment.

A wide variety of conflicting opinions on the relationship between orthodontics and TMD but dismissed many as they were the authors' personal opinions and were unsubstantiated.

Some studies indicate that orthodontic treatment is not responsible for creating a TMD either at the time of treatment or later, regardless of the orthodontic technique used, whether or not involving extractions and whether or not fixed or removable appliances were used. Moreover, other studies report that orthodontic treatment is not necessary to cure signs and symptoms of temporomandibular dysfunction but can form part of an overall treatment plan when appropriate.

Orthodontically treated patients, regardless of the type of therapeutic intervention, have no more and no fewer TMD symptoms than those found in the general population.

The literature therefore does not support a causative link between orthodontic treatment and TMD. The fact that a TMD may start soon after cessation of orthodontic treatment merely reflects the age of the patient. It is often in the late teens that a TMD would develop irrespective of whether or not orthodontic treatment had been undertaken and any link is usually coincidental. If a TMD develops during the course of treatment then this should be addressed in the usual manner and if the orthodontist is uneasy, then the patient should be referred for advice.

One consistent link between a basal bone and incisal relationship and risk of development of a TMD that the orthodontist should be aware of is the presence of an anterior open bite as this condition predisposes to development of a TMD in any case.

The widely accepted conclusion, therefore, is that orthodontic treatment neither causes nor cures TMD.

Restorative treatment, the dentist, and TMD

Can a dentist cause a TMD? Yes. This is not necessarily due to negligent treatment. Excessive or prolonged force on the mandible may play a role. Some individuals may develop symptoms from relatively simple dental treatment that would not lead to symptoms in others. Some are more susceptible than others. Placing a restoration which imbalances the rest of the occlusion may lead to a rapid onset of TMD symptoms and this is one of the very few occasions when direct occlusal adjustment may be a necessary part of treatment. Once the restoration feels comfortable, the TMD symptoms should resolve as long as there has not been a sufficient time lapse for them to become chronic.

If a dentist is undertaking a course of treatment in a hitherto asymptomatic patient and TMD signs or symptoms become evident then the situation should be re-evaluated. In the case of a click suddenly developing, one should be aware of the implications. The occlusion can alter rendering the final restoration occlusally inaccurate.

If the dentist is in the middle of a course of restorative treatment involving crowns or bridges and a click develops, placement of the final restoration should be delayed until it can be assessed whether the condition will resolve spontaneously or whether the patient should have the click treated. If the dentist ignores the change in clinical condition and proceeds with placement of the final restoration and the symptoms persist or worsen, he or she could be implicated in the perpetuation of the disorder.

If it is expected there is to be excessive force applied to the mandible or if the mouth is to be kept open for a prolonged period, then use a mouth prop and record this in the patient's notes. This is not only for patient comfort. When the mouth is stretched open, among others, the supra-hyoid, digastric, and lateral pterygoid muscles are active. The superior head of the lateral pterygoid is attached to the capsule and disc; the inferior head to the neck of the condyle. Prolonged contraction of this muscle can tend to pull the disc forwards. If a patient is biting on a prop, these muscles relax and closing muscles become active thereby causing less tension on the discal attachments. It is especially important to use a mouth prop in a known TMD patient. The dentist could be regarded as being at fault if this is ignored.

The use of a facebow and semi-adjustable articulators

A dentist can recognise the signs of occlusal instability not only by taking a thorough history and conducting a complete examination but also by reviewing diagnostic casts mounted on a semi-adjustable articulator in centric relation using a facebow transfer (Figure 14.8).

Although its use has not been yet supported by evidence-based studies, the use of a facebow is simple, quick, and highly recommended when accurate mounting of the casts is required. There appears to be no good reason for not using it.

When restoring anterior teeth, the facebow record provides considerable information for the dental technician and will help to obtain predictable results. If this vital record is not taken, the technician could mis-mount the cast, causing the final restorations to be inaccurate, because without a facebow determination of an occlusal plane could be guesswork.

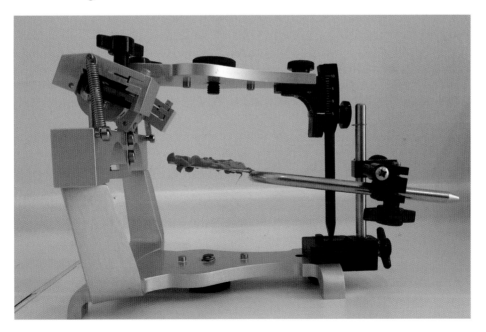

Figure 14.8 Facebow transfer on a semi-adjustable articulator for an accurate mounting of the casts. (M. Ziad Al-Ani, Robin J.M. Gray.)

Radiographs

Radiographs are rarely needed in TMD diagnosis or management. Radiographs should be reserved to confirm a clinical diagnosis if such confirmation is required, or alternatively to help formulate or change a treatment plan. Unless there are strong reasons that would indicate the need for such a special test, there is no justification for taking a radiograph. The same rationale applies to magnetic resonance imaging, computed tomography, and arthrography.

Further referral 13

It is important that you realise your limitations and the extent of your experience. If treatment is not progressing as you would expect, or if you feel that your patient's response to treatment is unusual or exaggerated, then immediately consider further referral for an expert opinion and make every effort to select a clinician with a special interest in TMDs. Historically, patients have been referred to the local oral surgery unit if there is no access to a dental school. In oral surgery units, it may be the case that a splint with no particular prescription will be prescribed. An alternative referral might be to a specialist orthodontist. It is readily accepted however that orthodontic treatment in isolation is not regarded as a treatment for a TMD. Collaboration with an orthodontist can be valuable, however, to alter localised interferences or to move a group of teeth to enable subsequent splint therapy to be more successful.

If the dentist feels treatment is outside their area of expertise, and if a patient is not referred promptly upon presentation of their symptoms, then there is a possibility that the symptoms will deteriorate, making subsequent treatment more difficult. An example is for a patient to present with a click which is left untreated and gradually becomes more intrusive and socially embarrassing as it becomes audible to others. This can on occasion progress to locking. The treatment of locking is less successful and more complex than the treatment for clicking. If the treatment had been instigated early on in the patient's course of symptoms, then they would have had a very much improved chance of successful management. The medico-legal implication of this situation is that the diagnosing dentist maintains a responsibility to ensure that prompt and appropriate referral takes place and must monitor their patient's progress.

Further Reading

Al-Ani Z. (2020). Occlusion and Temporomandibular Disorders: A Long-Standing Controversy in Dentistry. *Primary Dental Journal* 9: 43–48.

Al-Ani, Z. and Gray, R. (2007). TMD current concepts: 1. An update. *Dent Update* 34: 278–280, 282–4, 287–8.

Al-Ani, Z. and Gray, R. (2007). TMD current concepts: 2. Imaging and treatment options. An update. *Dent Update* 34: 356–358, 361–4, 367–70.

Clark, G.T., Tsukiyama, Y., Baba, K., and Watanable, T. (1999). Sixty-eight years of experimental occlusal interference studies: what have we learned? *J Prosthet Dent* 82: 704–713.

Durham, J., Aggarwal, V., Davies, S.J. et al. (2013). *Temporomandibular Disorders (TMDs): An Update and Management Guidance for Primary Care from the UK Specialist Interest Group in Orofacial Pain and TMDs (USOT)*, 22. England: *Royal College of Surgeons of England*. (Clinical Standard Series).

Davies, S. and Gray, R. (2000). Oral temazepam. *Br Dent J* 189: 467.

Durham, J., Exley, C., Wassell, R., and Steele, J.G. (2007). 'Management is a black art' – professional ideologies with respect to temporomandibular disorders. *Br Dent J* 202 (11): E29; discussion 682–3.

Foster, M.E., Gray, R.J., Davies, S.J., and Macfarlane, T.V. (2000). Therapeutic manipulation of the temporomandibular joint. *Br J Oral Maxillofac Surg* 38: 641–644.

Fricton, J. (2006). Current evidence providing clarity in management of temporomandibular disorders: summary of a systematic review of randomized clinical trials for intra-oral appliances and occlusal therapies. *J Evidence Based Dent Pract* 6: 48–52.

Gray, R.J. and Davies, S.J. (1997). Emergency treatment of acute temporomandibular disorders: Part I. *Dent Update* 24: 170–173.

Gray, R.J. and Davies, S.J. (1997). Emergency treatment of acute temporomandibular disorders: part II. *Dent Update* 24: 186–189.

Gray, R.J. and Davies, S.J. (2001). Occlusal splints and temporomandibular disorders: why, when, how? *Dent Update* 28: 194–199.

Gray, R.J., Davies, S.J., and Quayle, A.A. (1994). A clinical approach to temporomandibular disorders. 5. A clinical approach to treatment. *Br Dent J* 177: 101–106.

Gray, R.J., Davies, S.J., and Quayle, A.A. (1994). A clinical approach to temporomandibular disorders. 6. Splint therapy. *Br Dent J* 177: 135–142.

Gray, R.J., Davies, S.J., and Quayle, A.A. (1994). A clinical approach to temporomandibular disorders. 7. Treatment planning, general guidelines and case histories. *Br Dent J* 177: 171–178.

Gray, R.J., Davies, S.J., and Quayle, A.A. (1994). A clinical approach to temporomandibular disorders 9. The dentist and the specialist clinic. *Br Dent J* 177: 295–301.

Gray, R. and Al-Ani, Z. (2010). Risk management in clinical practice. Part 8. Temporomandibular disorders. *Br Dent J* 209: 433–449.

Gray, R. and Al-Ani, Z. (2013). Conservative temporomandibular disorder management: what DO I do? – frequently asked questions. *Dental Update* 40: 745–756.

Hasanain, F., Durham, J., Moufti, A. et al. (2009). Adapting the diagnostic definitions of the RDC/TMD to routine clinical practice: a feasibility study. *J Dent* 37: 955–962.

Hoad-Reddick, G. (2004). How relevant is counselling in relation to dentistry? *Br Dent J* 197: 9–14. quiz 50–1.

Koh, H. and Robinson, P.G. (2003). Occlusal adjustment for treating and preventing temporomandibular joint disorders. *Cochrane Database Syst Rev* 1 https://doi.org/10.1002/14651858.CD003812.

Luther, F. (2007). TMD and occlusion part I. Damned if we do? Occlusion: the interface of dentistry and orthodontics. *Br Dent J* 202 (1): E2; discussion 38–9.

Luther, F. (2007). TMD and occlusion part II. Damned if we don't? Functional occlusal problems: TMD epidemiology in a wider context. *Br Dent J* 202 (1): E3; discussion 38–9.

Okeson, J. (2019). *Management of Temporomandibular Disorders and Occlusion*, 8the. Mosby: Elsevier.

Milosevic, A. (2003). Occlusion: 2. Occlusal splints, analysis and adjustment. *Dent Update* 30: 416–422.

Nicolakis, P., Erdogmus, B., Kopf, A. et al. (2002). Effectiveness of exercise therapy in patients with myofascial pain dysfunction syndrome. *J Oral Rehabil* 29: 362–368.

O'Donovan, A.E., Ager, P.M., Davies, S.J., and Smith, P.W. (2003). An appraisal of the quality of referral letters from general dental practitioners to a temporomandibular disorder clinic. *Prim Dent Care* 10: 105–108.

Sidebottom, A.J. (2009). Current thinking in temporomandibular joint management. *Br J Oral Maxillofac Surg* 47: 91–94.

Tsukiyama, Y., Baba, K., and Clark, G.T. (2001). An evidence-based assessment of occlusal adjustment as a treatment for temporomandibular disorders. *J Prosthet Dent* 86: 57–66.

Wassell, R.W., Adams, N., and Kelly, P.J. (2004). Treatment of temporomandibular disorders by stabilising splints in general dental practice: results after initial treatment. *Br Dent J* 197: 35–41; discussion 31. quiz 50–1.

Wassell, R.W., Adams, N., and Kelly, P.J. (2006). The treatment of temporomandibular disorders with stabilizing splints in general dental practice: one-year follow-up. *J Am Dent Assoc* 137: 1089–1098. quiz 1168–9.

Evidence-based Dentistry

Al-Ani, M.Z., Davies, S.J., Gray, R.J.M. et al. (2004). Does splint therapy work for temporomandibular pain? *Evidence-Based Dent* 5: 65–66.

Al-Ani, Z., Gray, R.J., Davies, S.J. et al. (2005). Stabilization splint therapy for the treatment of temporomandibular myofascial pain: a systematic review. *J Dent Educ* 69: 1242–1250.

Al-Ani, Z., Davies, S., Sloan, P., and Gray, R. (2008). Change in the number of occlusal contacts following splint therapy in patients with a temporomandibular disorder (TMD). *Eur J Prosthodont Restor Dent* 16: 98–103.

Carlsson, G.E., Egermark, I., and Magnusson, T. (2003). Possible predictors of temporomandibular disorders. *Evidence-Based Dent* 4: 55.

Cascos-Romero, J., Vázquez-Delgado, E., Vázquez-Rodríguez, E., and Gay-Escoda, C. (2009). Inconsistent evidence for the use of tricyclic antidepressants in the treatment of temporomandibular joint disorders. *Evidence-Based Dent* 10: 56.

Crider, A.B. and Glaros, A.G. (2000). Efficacy of electromyographic treatment is supported for temporomandibular disorders. *Evidence-Based Dent* 2: 69.

De Boever, J.A., Nilner, M., Orthlieb, J.D., and Steenks, M.H. (2008). Educational committee of the european academy of craniomandibular disorders. Recommendations by the EACD for examination, diagnosis, and management of patients with temporomandibular disorders and orofacial pain by the general dental practitioner. *J Orofac Pain* 22: 268–278.

Farias-Neto, A., Dias, A., Miranda, B., and Oliveira, A. (2013). Face-bow transfer in prosthodontics: a systematic review of the literature. *J Oral Rehabil* 40 https://doi.org/10.1111/joor.12081.

Forssell, H., Kalso, E., Koskela, P. et al. (2000). Occlusal splints may be of benefit in TMD, but there is little evidence for the use of occlusal adjustment. *Evidence-Based Dent* 2: 67.

Fricton, J. (2006). Current evidence providing clarity in management of temporomandibular disorders: summary of a systematic review of randomized clinical trials for intra-oral appliances and occlusal therapies. *J Evidence Based Dent Pract* 6: 48–52.

Jakubowski A. (2010). The effects of manual therapy and exercise for adults with temporomandibular joint disorders compared to electrical modalities and exercise. *PT Critically Appraised Topics 2010*; Paper 13. http://commons.pacificu.edu/ptcats/13.

Kim, M.R., Graber, T.M., and Viana, M.A. (2002). Orthodontics and temporomandibular disorder: a meta-analysis. *Am J Orthod Dentofac Orthop* 121: 438–446.

Koh, H. and Robinson, P.G. (2003). There is no evidence to support use of occlusal adjustment for prevention or treatment of TMD. *Evidence-Based Dent* 4: 32.

Luther, F., Layton, S., and McDonald, F. (2016). Orthodontics for treating temporomandibular joint (TMJ) disorders. *Cochrane Database Syst Rev* 1: CD006541.

Manfredini, D., Bucci, M.B., Montagna, F., and Guari, L. (2011). Temporomandibular disorders assessment: medicolegal considerations in the evidence-based era. *J Oral Rehabil* 38: 101–119.

Manfredini, D., Lombardo, L., and Siciliani, G. (2017). Temporomandibular disorders and dental occlusion. A systematic review of association studies: end of an era? *J Oral Rehabil* 44: 908–923.

Michelotti, A. and Iodice, G. (2010). The role of orthodontics in temporomandibular disorders. *J Oral Rehabil* 37: 411–429.

Minakuchi, H., Kuboki, T., Malsuka, Y. et al. (2002). Patients with anterior disk displacement improve with minimal treatment. *Evidence-Based Dent* 3: 69.

Mujakperuo, H.R., Watson, M., Morrison, R., and Macfarlane, T.V. (2010). Pharmacological interventions for pain in patients with temporomandibular disorders. *Cochrane Database Syst Rev* 10: CD004715.

Chapter 15

You and the Lawyer

We live in a litigious era, which means that as clinicians we also practise in a litigious era. This does not mean that you must adopt a litigation-based philosophy in your treatment planning, as this would not be in your patient's best interests. What it does mean, however, is that you must keep contemporaneous records that are accurate, precise, and indisputable. You must discuss all treatment options with your patient, however inappropriate you may feel that they are, giving you reasons for your advice. You must not project yourself as having skills or training that you do not possess. You must employ evidence-based treatments. We consider three different case scenarios.

Case scenario 1: note and record-keeping

Gray & Al-Ani Solicitors
101 Manchester Road
Manchester
M1 2XY

Our Ref: SSDAB/SMI111-01

Jones Dental Care
162 Union Road
Manchester M1 3AB
Dear Sirs

Re: Our Client/Your patient: Joy Smith d.o.b. 10.10.1951
Address: 13 Brides Drive Manchester M1 12CD

Temporomandibular Disorders: A Problem-Based Approach, Second Edition. M. Ziad Al-Ani and Robin J.M. Gray.
© 2021 M. Ziad Al-Ani and Robin J.M. Gray. Published 2021 by John Wiley & Sons Ltd.
Companion Website: www.wiley.com/go/al-ani/temporomandibular-disorders-2e

We are instructed to act on behalf of Mrs Smith in connection with a claim for damages arising out of an accident in which she was involved.

We should be grateful if you would kindly provide us with copies of Mrs Smith's entire dental notes, records, correspondence, radiological images, test results, investigation reports, referrals, etc.

We enclose our client's written authority for this purpose and confirm that we shall be responsible for your fees in relation to this request up to a maximum of £50.00.

We also confirm that, as far as we are aware, these records are not required in relation to any litigation against yourself or your practice.

We look forward to hearing from you within 14 days.

Yours faithfully

Authority to release dental notes and records

Our Ref: SSDAB/SMI111-01

Jones Dental Care
162 Union Road
Manchester M1 3AB

Dear Sirs

I, Joy Smith of 13 Brides Drive, Manchester M1 12CD, hereby authorise the release of all of my Dental Records, Notes, Memoranda and X-rays to my solicitors:

Gray & Al-Ani Solicitors
101 Manchester Road
Manchester M1 2XY

The release of these notes relates to a claim for damages arising out of an accident in which I was involved on the 23rd April and I confirm that they are not required in relation to any litigation against Jones Dental Care.

Signed . . . .

Dated . . . .

You know that you are duty bound to provide the records within a certain period of time that is deemed to be reasonable. If retrieval of your records will take longer than the suggested time, it is your responsibility to contact the solicitors to advise them that you cannot comply with the timescale that they have set and agree a more realistic timescale.

You ask your practice manager to download the notes from the computer and provide you with all hard copy notes that you had kept before your practice was computerised. You are in the unfortunate situation of not having any idea about the injuries, the details of the accident, or the date.

When your manager brings you the notes, she says that she cannot find any radiographs because they appear to have been lost. There are no radiographs scanned into the computer system. You saw Mrs Smith on only three occasions and have only a vague recollection of her. You have no hard copy notes and your computerised printout gives only the barest details of examinations and treatment actually completed. You had not recorded an examination of her articulatory system.

You had seen her on three occasions at approximately yearly intervals and the last time you saw her was over a year ago. Your initial examination contained some scanty details about her presenting complaints and expectations and you recorded the fact that she was not happy with her previous dentist. She was not a regular attender.

You had recorded a baseline charting recording her missing teeth and existing restorations and you had completed a BPE chart. She had plaque and calculus lingual to her lower anteriors, but the rest of the intraoral and extraoral examination boxes had not been completed. Two small restorations needed replacing due to recurrent caries. You took bite-wing radiographs (subsequently lost). You completed the two restorations without incident. She attended the hygienist.

She did not return for over 12 months and then again 12 months later. No further clinical records had been completed apart from an examination and hygienist referral on both occasions. No further radiographs were taken.

You phoned the solicitors and were advised that her problem was a jaw problem after a road traffic accident.

Due to the inadequacy of your record–keeping, you were not able to furnish the solicitors with any useful information, but you did return what you had. You received a personal phone call from one of the solicitors requesting further information as to whether Mrs Smith did have a pre-existing jaw condition. You were unable to help.

This situation is all too familiar in clinical practice. It is your responsibility to keep accurate and complete records, take radiographs according to (IR(ME)R) 2018 regulations, and keep an up-to-date periodontal index. You are required to undertake a complete examination of your patients at the initial consultation and at each subsequent 6-monthly or 12-monthly examination visit.

Many practices are computerised so it is very easy to merely tick boxes on a computer proforma and complete an absolute minimum of additional entries.

Letters such as this from solicitors may arrive many months or even years after you last saw a patient. You are leaving yourself vulnerable if a situation such as this does arise.

Case scenario 2: a medical report request

You are a well-known dentist in your neighbourhood with many years of clinical experience. After qualifying you spent 18 months as a house officer in oral and maxillofacial surgery. You receive a letter from instructing solicitors asking if you are prepared to produce a report for one of their clients who had had an accident involving 'dental injuries'. She lives close to your practice and because of personal circumstances is unwilling to travel far. Her usual dentist did not feel that he had the experience to help.

You feel flattered and readily agree to do this.

Do you get enough information? Have you got the necessary experience?

A large bundle of notes is delivered to your practice containing the client's contact details, a very brief description of the circumstances of the accident, and a letter of instruction that outlines your duties and responsibilities to the court and a suggested declaration for you to sign.

What will you receive?

A letter of instruction that contains a paragraph stating:

Following examination of our client we will require your report to deal with the following specific points, in addition to providing the usual information:

1. *Did our client have a pre-existing temporomandibular dysfunction?*
2. *If so to what extent?*
3. *If the answers to 1 and 2 above are in the negative, do you feel that the injuries claimed by the patient would have initiated her current symptoms?*
4. *In the event that she is not fully recovered, how long do you consider it will take her to recover to the pre-accident state?*
5. *In the event that you consider our client did have a pre-existing condition, have her symptoms been exacerbated by the accident. Do you believe that treatment is appropriate? If so please specify giving costs.*
6. *Please comment on our client's ability to return to work.*
7. *Please comment on what psychological stress you feel that she may have suffered.*

You will receive a quantity of notes

The bundle of records included the following:

- The general medical practitioners records
- Her dental records

- Her dental hospital records
- Her Royal Infirmary records
- Her records from a walk-in NHS centre.

The brief description of the incident recorded that she had been on a night out with some friends and she alleged that she had been assaulted by her boyfriend. She received two blows to the face. She was not rendered unconscious but she felt that she might have broken her jaw. She went to an NHS walk-in centre who were unable to help and they referred her to the Royal Infirmary. No radiographs were taken because it was felt that she had not broken her jaw, but by this stage, she could not open her mouth because her jaw was very stiff and her face was bruised and swollen. She was also aware of having broken some teeth.

You felt that it was within your area of competence to provide a report and you saw her at your surgery for an examination. Her relationship with her boyfriend had been tempestuous and he had threatened her in the past, but had never actually struck her. She only had a very scanty recollection of events on the night because they had been out 'celebrating'. She was a poor historian and frequently contradicted herself.

The alleged assault had happened nine months previously. She said that she had acute symptoms from her left jaw joint and left earache for two to three weeks. This had gradually lessened but had never gone away completely.

Her complaints were audible clicking from her left jaw joint, and pain on chewing and when opening wide. She had not experienced any locking. She said that she had chipped two or three teeth when she was struck but these had been minor chips and had been repaired adequately by her general dental practitioner. She was concerned about her jaw and was pursuing a claim against her former boyfriend.

When you started your clinical examination there were one or two features that you found surprising. She opened normally to over 40 mm on some occasions but on other occasions she was only opening to 25 mm. She said her jaw 'would not go' although she had earlier told you that she had no locking. When she opened her mouth she sometimes had a straight pathway of opening but not on other occasions. When you listened for joint sounds, you could hear a very soft occasional click but not the loud audible click that she described. When you examined the lateral pterygoid muscle under resistance, the area of tenderness to which she pointed was under the angle of the mandible, not the preauricular region. She said that she had never had a previous temporomandibular disorder (TMD).

Let us go back now to your letter of instruction and the bundle of documents.

Doctor's records

You were provided with her general medical practitioner's records. These dated back over 12 years and in these records there were repeated references to jaw pain and clicking. She was a very frequent attender at her doctors.

Dentist's records

Her general dental practitioner's records had been extremely well kept. She had been a regular patient and there were recurrent records of a TMD with a reduced range of mouth opening, TMJ and muscle tenderness, and intermittent clicking. He had last seen her two months before the injury.

Walk-in centre records

The walk-in centre records recorded that she had attended late one night, stating that she had been assaulted. She had some facial swelling and bruising and was advised to attend the accident and emergency department. It was recorded she smelled of alcohol and her speech was slurred.

Royal Infirmary records

Her local Royal Infirmary notes recorded that no radiographs were taken and she did not have any fracture of the bony structures. She was advised to see her dentist in relation to the chipped teeth.

Dental hospital records

She saw her dentist two days after the assault and he referred her to the dental hospital for radiographs. There were various mentions in the dental hospital records that her symptoms varied surprisingly. Physiotherapy had no effect. Sometimes she complained of severe pain but clinical findings did not substantiate this. She was provided with a soft vacuum formed splint which she did not wear. She failed two further appointments.

Your report

Considering the specific points that the solicitor has asked you to deal with, we can refer back to these numbered points and answer them in
turn:

1. You would have to reply honestly that, in spite of her adamant report of no pre-existing condition, there is substantial evidence that she had a long-standing TMD.
2. List her symptoms from her doctor's and dentist's notes with dates.

3. Make the statement that there are discrepancies in the patient's report, your clinical findings and other records. It is up to the court to decide fact.

4. You cannot commit yourself as to how long her symptoms will be present. A patient's response to treatment is individual. Suggest that she has treatment done and is then reassessed.

5. Suggest a treatment plan with costs and approximate dates.
6. This is outwith your area of expertise. You are not qualified to answer this; the person to do so would be an occupational therapist – not you.

7. This is outwith your area of expertise; a clinical psychologist or psychiatrist should see the patient and provide a report – not you.

In retrospect it might have been better for you to decline the instructions and not to have agreed to prepare a report at all. You have a patient who may be lying. Throughout this report you are making comments that you are not qualified to deliver. You must be prepared to stand up and be cross-examined about your report. Your own history of oral and maxillofacial surgery was only an 18-month house officer job. Although you may have had experience of dealing with patients with TMD in general practice, you had not made this an area of special interest. You must never comment on areas outside your area of expertise.

Case scenario 3: a disgruntled patient

You have been treating Miss Winston for several years. You have always had a fairly 'fragile' relationship with her because she does not accept treatment readily as she is very nervous. You had always felt that she was a habitual complainer!

She attended some months ago complaining of pain from an upper left first molar. You removed a restoration and replaced it with a crown. After the crown was fitted she said her bite did not feel quite right but it appeared acceptable to you.

When she was on her way home from the surgery she heard a loud crack from her lower left first molar, which was heavily restored. She phoned and you saw her the following day, by which time she was in severe pain from the lower tooth. You saw that a cusp of the lower molar had fractured, which you removed, and saw that there was a pulp exposure. You pulp capped this with calcium hydroxide and dressed the tooth, telling her that the symptoms would now settle. The symptoms did not in fact settle and after repeated reviews you eventually suggested an extraction. This she agreed to and the tooth was removed. You heard no more about the matter until 3 months later when you received the following letter. This was accompanied by the authority to release dental notes and records signed by the patient.

Gray & Al-Ani Solicitors
   101 Manchester Road
   Manchester M1 2XY
Our Ref: SSDAB/SMI111-01

Jones Dental Care
162 Union Road
Manchester M1 3AB
Dear Sirs

Re: Our Client/Your patient: Joy Smith d.o.b. 10.10.1951
Address: 13 Brides Drive Manchester M1 12CD

We have been instructed by the above named, who we understand is a patient of your dental practice. She is considering pursuing a claim for dental negligence.

Please forward all of her clinical records, X-rays and correspondence forthwith.

Yours sincerely

You obviously must comply forthwith with these instructions and provide all the details that you have been asked for.

It is essential at this stage that you inform your indemnity protection society or defence union, which will want a full report on the sequence of events in chronological order and all other relevant records. Send only photocopies of your records to the requesting solicitor. At this stage do not contact the patient. Acknowledge receipt of the solicitor's letter. Wait to hear from your indemnity society.

The next correspondence that you receive contains further documents from Mrs Smith's solicitors.

Particulars of claim

1. At all relevant times the claimant was a patient of the defendant who practises as a dentist in the Jones Dental Care practice in Manchester.
2. The defendant inappropriately advised the claimant that she would require a crown at her UL6.
3. After the procedure was finished the claimant felt that something was not right with her teeth in that the crown was high on the bite.
4. The claimant later heard a loud crack in her mouth and felt that part of her lower tooth had been pushed into her gum. She was in immediate and severe pain.
5. The claimant returned to see the Defendant. She was experiencing extreme pain.
6. It was noted that the LL6 had fractured.
7. The claimant's LL6 was extracted.
8. The claimant has now developed a click in her left jaw joint, cannot open her mouth normally and has left facial pain.
9. The defendant's treatment of the claimant was negligent.

Particulars of negligence

The defendant was negligent in that he:

Incorrectly advised the claimant that she would require a crown at UL6 when there was no clinical need for such treatment.

At no time were any other treatment options discussed with the claimant apart from extraction of LL6.

Caused the claimant to develop a temporomandibular disorder.

By reason of the matters aforesaid, the claimant has suffered pain and injury and has sustained loss and damage.

Particulars of injury

As a result of the negligence alleged herein, the claimant developed pain and suffering related to the fracture of LL6 and the tooth had to be extracted. At no stage was the possibility of root canal treatment discussed. There was no mention of bridging and there was no mention of replacement of the fractured tooth by means of an osseo-integrated implant. She has also developed a temporomandibular dysfunction and facial pain that is continuing to cause her discomfort.

The claimant will require an osseo-integrated implant which will be restored with a crown once it has integrated with the bone. The crown will have to be replaced every 10 years. She would require either a general anaesthetic or a local anaesthetic with intravenous sedation for this procedure because of her ongoing facial pain, anxiety, and her TMD.

The prognosis is good in relation to the osseo-integrated implant but is guarded in relation to her TMD.

The claimant will rely upon medical reports of Mr Smith and Dr Brown, copies of which are served herewith and such further evidences as may become available to her.

The claimant will claim interest if such damages may be awarded pursuant to Section 69 of the County Courts Act 1984 at such rate and for such a period as the court thinks fit.

The claimant claims damages including a claim for personal injuries in excess of £1000.00 but with the total claim limited to £50 000.00 and interest thereon as aforesaid.

Do not underestimate the anxiety and stress that the next few months will cause. Let us look at the facts.

You fitted a crown to the UL6 for this lady and she states that you did not discuss fully with her the other treatment options for the tooth. She is now claiming that this crown was not clinically necessary. You did not examine the occlusion closely enough when the crown was fitted to the extent that she was able to detect that her bite was incorrect. You did not adjust the occlusion. When you noted that the lower first molar was fractured with a small pulp exposure, you did not proceed to root canal therapy, you continually redressed the tooth until irreversible pulpitis and pulp necrosis occurred. You did not attempt to extirpate the pulp yourself. You did not refer her for specialist endodontic treatment.

From her statement, it appears that there was no discussion of replacement of the gap left by extraction of this tooth. She appears to have developed a TMD having previously been symptom free and she attributes this to your treatment.

Her claim is quite correct and has merit. Your position is difficult to defend.

This is an extreme case scenario but not an infrequent one. The most important thing when dealing with patients is always to treat with their best interests at heart.

What generally leads to cases such as this arriving on the desks of solicitors is a breakdown in communication. It is essential that you maintain communication with your patients at all time and do not dismiss them as 'complainers'.

Never be tempted to alter, amend, add to or remove entries in patient records. Not only is this dishonest but it is detectable, and discovery of any attempt at fraud will be dealt with harshly.

If you are ever involved in dealing with solicitors, the first people you **must** inform are your indemnity society or defence union. This is their job and you will find their supportive advice and practical help invaluable.

Further Reading

Al-Ani, Z. and Gray, R. (2007). TMD current concepts: 2. Imaging and treatment options. An update. *Dent Update* 34: 356–358, 361–4, 367–70.

GDC Standards for the Dental Team. 2013 Available at: https://www.gdc-uk.org/information-standards-guidance/standards-and-guidance/standards-for-the-dental-team/

Gelbier, S., Wright, D., and Bishop, M. (2001). Ethics and dentistry: 2. Ethics and risk management. *Dent Update* 28: 524.

Gray, R. and Al-Ani, Z. (2010). Risk management in clinical practice. Part 8. Temporomandibular disorders. *Br Dent J* 209: 433–449.

The Ionising Radiation (Medical Exposure) (Amendment) Regulations 2018. Available at: https://www.cqc.org.uk/guidance-providers/ionising-radiation/ionising-radiation-medical-exposure-regulations-irmer

Chapter 16

The Referral Letter

 13 This is not meant to be a condescending section. Referral letters vary from the very helpful to the valueless.

All too often referral letters are received that say in their entirety: 'This patient has a TMD; please see and treat'. Sometimes even the patient's contact details are missing. This is of no value to either the patient or the treating clinician.

This is a template for the details that an ideal referral letter should contain. Some of the details will not always be relevant but the referral letter should not be regarded as 'refer and forget'. You are asking a specialist to help you in your patient's management. This might be a brief interlude in your patient's history, but from your point of view you may be entering long-term supervision of a chronic problem that might need to be revisited at intervals, so you need to understand the specialist's philosophy and match it to your patient's needs.

Details

 Obvious details to include are the patient's personal and contact details. Full name, address, date of birth, day time, evening and, if acceptable to the patient, mobile telephone numbers.

History

 A brief history of the patient's complaints is invaluable. Remember that some signs and symptoms come and go in patients with a temporomandibular disorder (TMD) but it is useful to have a chronological order of what the patient has been experiencing. For instance:

Temporomandibular Disorders: A Problem-Based Approach, Second Edition. M. Ziad Al-Ani and Robin J.M. Gray.
© 2021 M. Ziad Al-Ani and Robin J.M. Gray. Published 2021 by John Wiley & Sons Ltd.
Companion Website: www.wiley.com/go/al-ani/temporomandibular-disorders-2e

- Did pain precede a click or did a click precede pain?
- Has the patient ever had locking?
- Is the range of movement restricted?
- Are symptoms overall worsening or improving?
- Are symptoms worse at any particular time of day?
- What is the precise location of the pain?
- How severe is it?
- Is the patient aware of any contributing factors such as bruxism or clenching?

Remember that you know your patients better than the clinician who will see them for the first time. You know their treatment expectations and their response to treatment. You may be referring this patient only because you have undertaken all the normally accepted treatments and the symptoms have either not improved or gradually got worse. This is useful information to impart.

Has the patient been compliant with the treatment that you have suggested?

It is useful to know whether you have provided a splint but you suspect that the patient hasn't worn it. You might have tried to arrange for physiotherapy but the patient did not turn up. You may have suggested some anti-inflammatory medication but the patient declined to take it.

Medical and social history

Give a brief synopsis of the patient's relevant medical history, this has obvious implications. Outline any social factors that you may think are relevant; it might be useful to know if the patient is being referred privately, if he or she has private health insurance. Some treatments can be very expensive and it is better for the treating clinician to know this rather than embarrass the patient by involving him or her in potentially expensive investigations or treatment. Give details of any other specific problems that you feel may be of interest to the treating clinician. Patients, when seen in a strange environment for the first time by somebody they don't know, are often anxious and nervous, so it might be useful if you suggest that they write down some of the important facts and dates before they see the specialist; tell them also to make a note of any questions that they may wish to ask. If appropriate, advise the treating clinician of this in your letter. It is often very useful for the specialist to have such personal comments photocopied and kept in the patient's notes, if they are in agreement with this being done.

Request

 Finally, please ask the treating clinician what you want them to do. Do you want them to evolve a treatment plan that is practice based; one that you can undertake yourself in your own practice, or do you want them to undertake all further treatment in relation to the TMD?

Remember that this may include not only all arrangements relevant to the TMD, such as splint therapy and arranging for physiotherapy, but also in some cases extensive occlusal rehabilitation or other restorative treatment. Some patients referred to a TMD clinic have significant occlusal wear, attrition, or tooth surface loss. Is this in your remit to restore or do you wish the treating clinician to do it or arrange for it?

All this information will help enormously in what can sometimes be quite a short examination and interview time once introductions have been made and the patient seated comfortably.

Sometimes when patient's symptoms start after an incident, such as a road traffic accident or assault, he or she finds it quite upsetting to relive the situation and this can be avoided if handled correctly and sympathetically. Giving this advanced knowledge reassures the patient that you are involved in the case and know something about it and are interested.

Referring a patient for specialist examination or treatment does not mean 'refer and forget'. It is the responsibility of the referring clinician to monitor the patient's progress and if they or the patient are not satisfied with the progress, to undertake appropriate re-referral. It is not common in the management of patients with temporomandibular disorders for patients to be referred to 'specialists' only to be offered potent drug regimes, inappropriate splints, or on occasion surgery.

Further Reading

Anastassaki, A. and Magnusson, T. (2004). Patients referred to a specialist clinic because of suspected temporomandibular disorders: a survey of 3194 patients in respect of diagnoses, treatments, and treatment outcome. *Acta Odontol Scand* 62: 183–192.

Gray, R.J., Davies, S.J., and Quayle, A.A. (1994). A clinical approach to temporomandibular disorders 9. The dentist and the specialist clinic. *Br Dent J* 177: 295–301.

O'Donovan, A.E., Ager, P.M., Davies, S.J., and Smith, P.W. (2003). An appraisal of the quality of referral letters from general dental practitioners to a temporomandibular disorder clinic. *Prim Dent Care* 10: 105–108.

Chapter 17

How to Make a Splint ⑤7

How do you make a stabilisation splint?

Upper and lower models of the patient's dental arches are cast from alginate impressions using Die-stone.

Facebow registration

This relates the upper model of the dental arch to the hinges of the articulator in the same spatial relationship as exists between the maxillary teeth and the temporomandibular joints (TMJs). This helps to determine that, during construction of the splint, any opening or closing of the semi-adjustable articulator occurs along the same arc as in the mouth (Figure 17.1).

Armamentarium (Figure 17.2)

- Earbow
- Bitefork and vertical transfer jig assembly

Reference plane locator

- Marker pen
- Rigid bite registration material or beauty wax.

Locating and marking a reference point on the patient's face

An anterior reference point, along with the other two posterior points, needs to be established first for an accurate facebow record. The position

Temporomandibular Disorders: A Problem-Based Approach, Second Edition. M. Ziad Al-Ani and Robin J.M. Gray.
© 2021 M. Ziad Al-Ani and Robin J.M. Gray. Published 2021 by John Wiley & Sons Ltd.
Companion Website: www.wiley.com/go/al-ani/temporomandibular-disorders-2e

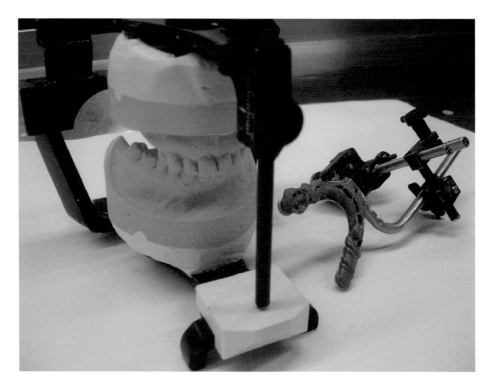

Figure 17.1 Facebow registration has been used to relate the upper model of the dental arch to the hinges of the articulator. (M. Ziad Al-Ani, Robin J.M. Gray.)

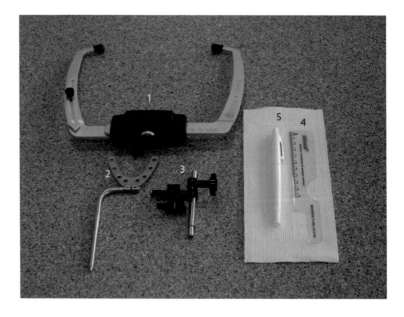

Figure 17.2 Earbow and accessories needed for facebow registration: (1) Slidematic U-shape earbow; (2) dentate bitefork; (3) transfer jig; (4) reference plane locator; and (5) marker pen. (M. Ziad Al-Ani, Robin J.M. Gray.)

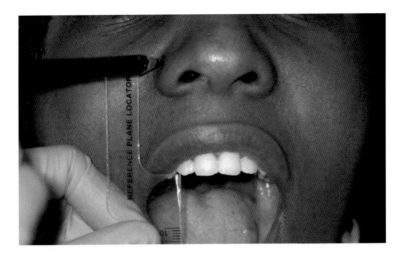

Figure 17.3 Marking the anterior reference point. (M. Ziad Al-Ani, Robin J.M. Gray.)

of the anterior reference point is measured 43 mm from the incisal edge of the central or lateral incisor, towards the inner corner of the eye. The notched-out area of the 'reference plane locator' is used to make this measurement. Mark the anterior reference point on the patient's face using a marker (Figure 17.3).

Taking the facebow registration (assembling the earbow on the patient)

Load the upper surface of the bitefork with two thicknesses of beauty wax. A rigid silicone bite registration material may also be used as bite fork recording material (Figure 17.4).

Soften the wax to a very soft consistency in warm water or over an open flame. With the bitefork arm projecting to the patient's right, place it on to the patient's upper teeth, aligning midline to obtain a light indexing impression of the maxillary teeth. Stabilise this by instructing the patient to hold it steady using the thumbs. Let the material harden before proceeding (Figures 17.5 and 17.6).

Loosen the centre wheel on the earbow and loosen the finger screws on the transfer jig.

Slide the transfer jig onto the bitefork arm and guide the earbow into the patient's ears with their help. Pull the earbow together and tighten the centre wheel, ensuring even placement in both ear canals (Figure 17.7).

Raise or lower the bow so that the pointer aligns with the anterior reference point on the patient's face. You can also look through a slot in the bow to verify this. Engage the transfer jig in the earbow and tighten finger screws 1 and 2 on the transfer jig, being careful not to torque the earbow.

Always ensure that the numbers '1' and '2' are the correct way up and facing you (Figure 17.8).

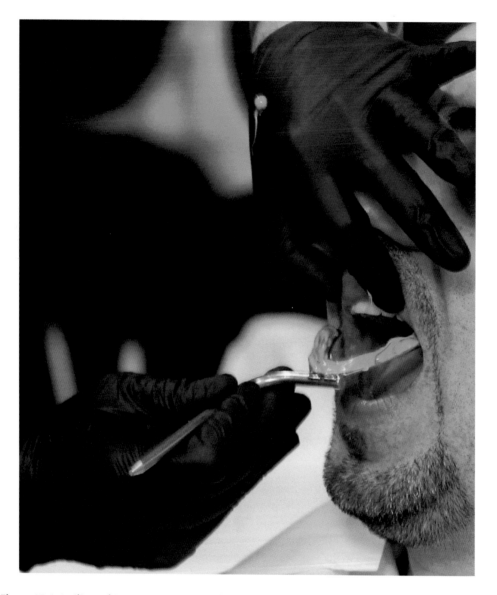

Figure 17.4 A silicone bite registration material can be used as bite fork recording medium. (M. Ziad Al-Ani, Robin J.M. Gray.)

Have the patient stand and, looking at the patient from the front, verify that the bow is horizontal to the horizon and the patient's pupils. Some facebow systems include a bubble level which will help in this verification (Figure 17.9).

Adjust as necessary and retighten finger screws 1 and 2 as necessary (Figure 17.10).

Loosen the centre screw on the earbow; slide open and remove the entire earbow assembly, transfer jig, and bitefork from the patient (Figure 17.11).

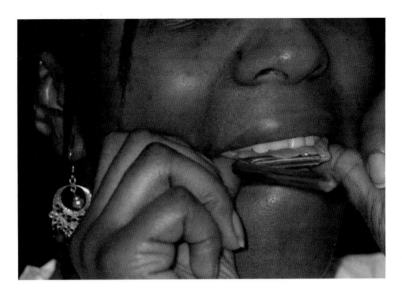

Figure 17.5 The bitefork is placed on to patient's upper teeth and stabilised by patient's thumbs. (M. Ziad Al-Ani, Robin J.M. Gray.)

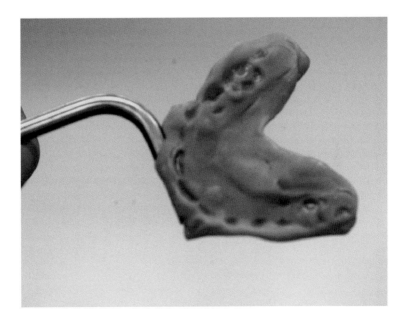

Figure 17.6 Light indexing impression of the maxillary teeth on the bite fork. (M. Ziad Al-Ani, Robin J.M. Gray.)

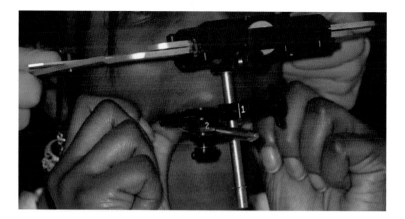

Figure 17.7 The earbow is guided into the patient's ears. (M. Ziad Al-Ani, Robin J.M. Gray.)

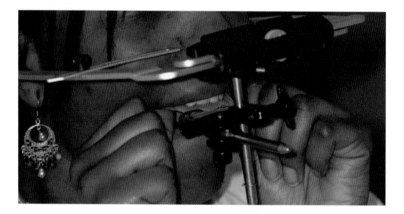

Figure 17.8 The pointer is aligned with anterior reference point on the patient's face. (M. Ziad Al-Ani, Robin J.M. Gray.)

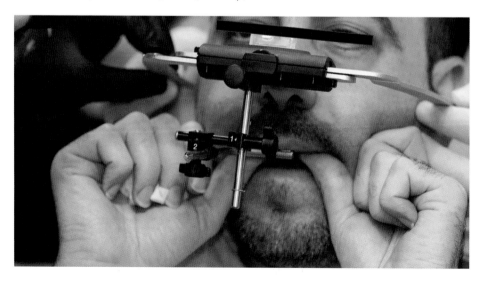

Figure 17.9 Looking at the patient from the front, verify that the bow is horizontal to the horizon and the patient's pupils. A bubble level can help in this verification. (M. Ziad Al-Ani, Robin J.M. Gray.)

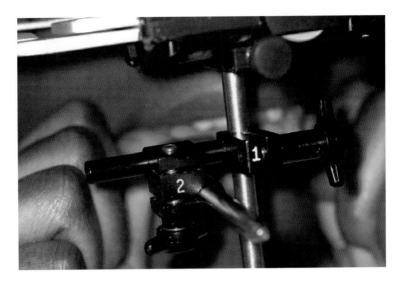

Figure 17.10 Finger screws 1 and 2 are securely tightened before removing the earbow. (M. Ziad Al-Ani, Robin J.M. Gray.)

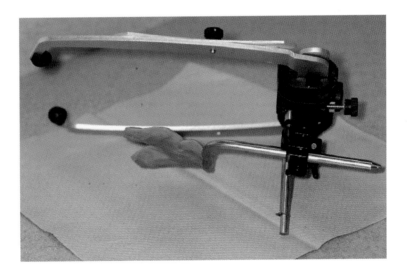

Figure 17.11 The earbow assembly, transfer jig, and bitefork are removed from patient. (M. Ziad Al-Ani, Robin J.M. Gray.)

Detach the earbow from the transfer jig assembly. Carefully tighten finger screws 1 and 2, making sure not to torque or change the transfer jig assembly (Figure 17.12).

Disinfect the transfer jig assembly and send it to the laboratory for mounting.

Centric relation record

A centric relation registration is taken by inducing relaxation of the masticatory muscles through the gentle arcing of the mandible up and

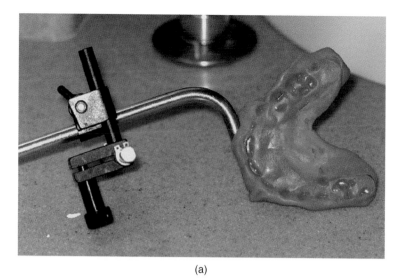

(a)

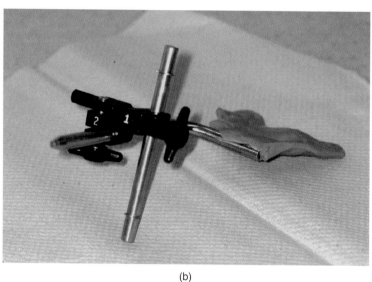

(b)

Figure 17.12 (a) Transfer jig after detachment from the earbow; (b) screws 1 and 2 should be tightened before transferring to the laboratory. (M. Ziad Al-Ani, Robin J.M. Gray.)

down, along the closing arc of the terminal hinge axis, using gentle bimanual manipulation while the patient is supine. It has been suggested that the patient's mandible describes a perfect arc during manipulation, which gives the operator the confidence that the terminal hinge axis of the mandible has been found (Figure 17.13).

A small quantity of warm, soft, and greenstick impression compound is placed over the palatal and incisal surfaces of the upper anterior teeth during this manipulation, until the lower anterior teeth make indentations in the material. This is used as a template when it has cooled

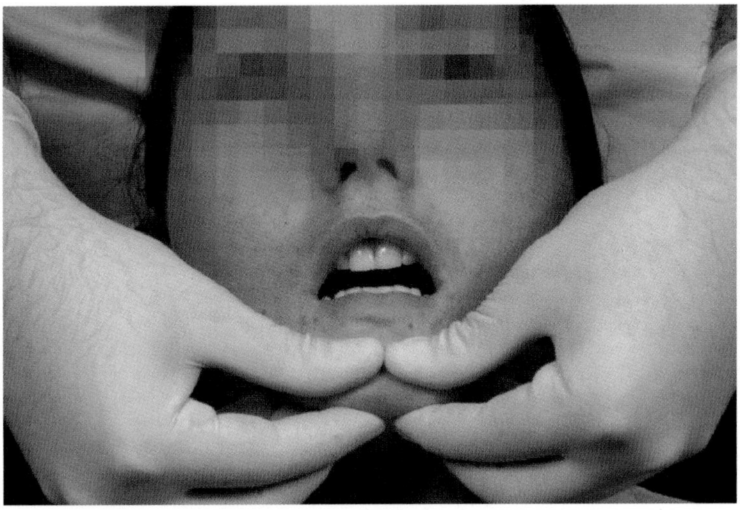

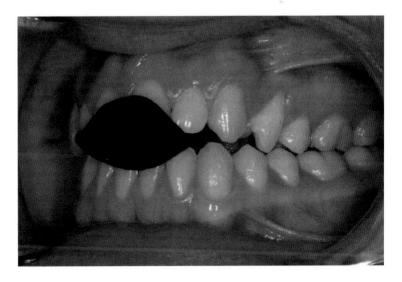

Figure 17.13 Passive manipulation of the mandible of a supine patient used for achieving centric relation. (M. Ziad Al-Ani, Robin J.M. Gray.)

and hardened to assist the patient in reproducibly closing into centric relation (Figure 17.14).

A suitable bite registration material (polyvinylsiloxane) is then syringed into the interocclusal posterior gap bilaterally; once this has hardened, the greenstick is subsequently replaced by a further mix of bite registration material on the anterior teeth, using the set material on the posterior teeth as a template to obtain a full, single, horseshoe–shoe centric relation registration (Figures 17.15 and 17.16).

Figure 17.14 Greenstick impression compound used as a template into which the patient is able to close in centric relation after manipulation of the mandible to centric relation. (M. Ziad Al-Ani, Robin J.M. Gray.)

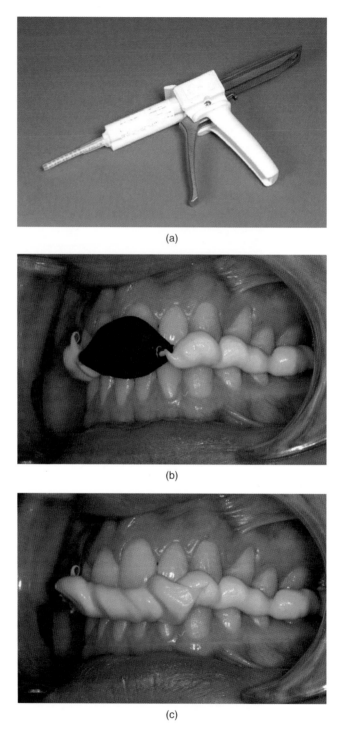

(a)

(b)

(c)

Figure 17.15 A suitable bite registration material is syringed between the posterior teeth, with the greenstick impression compound used as a template for achieving a complete centric relation. (M. Ziad Al-Ani, Robin J.M. Gray.)

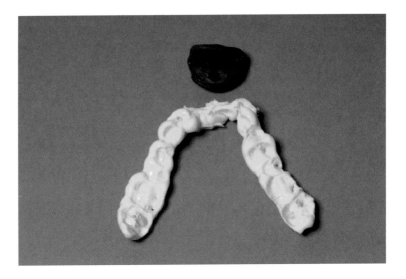

Figure 17.16 The completed centric relation bite registration with the impression compound template, which is subsequently discarded. (M. Ziad Al-Ani, Robin J.M. Gray.)

This centric relation registration with the impressions and facebow transfer jig record is sent to the laboratory, and the models of the arches are mounted in the semi-adjustable articulator (Figures 17.17 and 17.18).

Adequate relief of undercuts and initial polishing are carried out in the laboratory to ensure easy seating of the splint (Figures 17.19).

Fitting a stabilisation splint

It will take approximately an hour to fit and balance the splint in the patient's mouth. The splint will be delivered from the laboratory with adequate relief of undercuts to ensure easy seating. The stabilisation splint should be relined with autopolymerising acrylic, intraorally at the chairside, to provide good and positive retention (Figure 17.20).

During relining, the acrylic is applied to the fitting surface of the splint which is then placed on to the teeth and fully seated. The splint must be removed from the mouth before the acrylic has fully set and, when it has set, any excess is removed using an acrylic trimmer in a straight handpiece. It should then be tried to ensure that it is not too tight but has good retention (Figure 17.21).

Central relation occlusion (CRO) is then established by adjusting the splint, after marking the occlusal contacts using articulating paper until a balanced series of posterior centric stops has been produced. During this procedure, the splint is inserted into the mouth, and the patient's mandible is gently tapped up and down with the articulating paper interposed between the surface of the splint and the opposing teeth. The splint is then removed and any necessary adjustments are made (Figure 17.22).

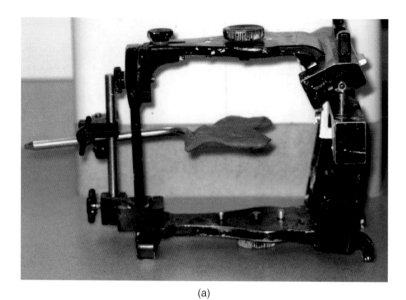

(a)

(b)

Figure 17.17 (a) The earbow transfer jig is transferred to a semi-adjustable articulator; (b) the upper model is positioned on the articulator using the transfer jig record. (M. Ziad Al-Ani, Robin J.M. Gray.)

Balancing commences by ensuring that the opposing canines touch in centric relation. A balanced occlusion should be provided between the splint and one cusp tip of every opposing tooth, distally from the canines. Repetitive adjustments of the splint are made after marking the occlusal contacts with thin articulating paper, until a full range of centric stops has been achieved.

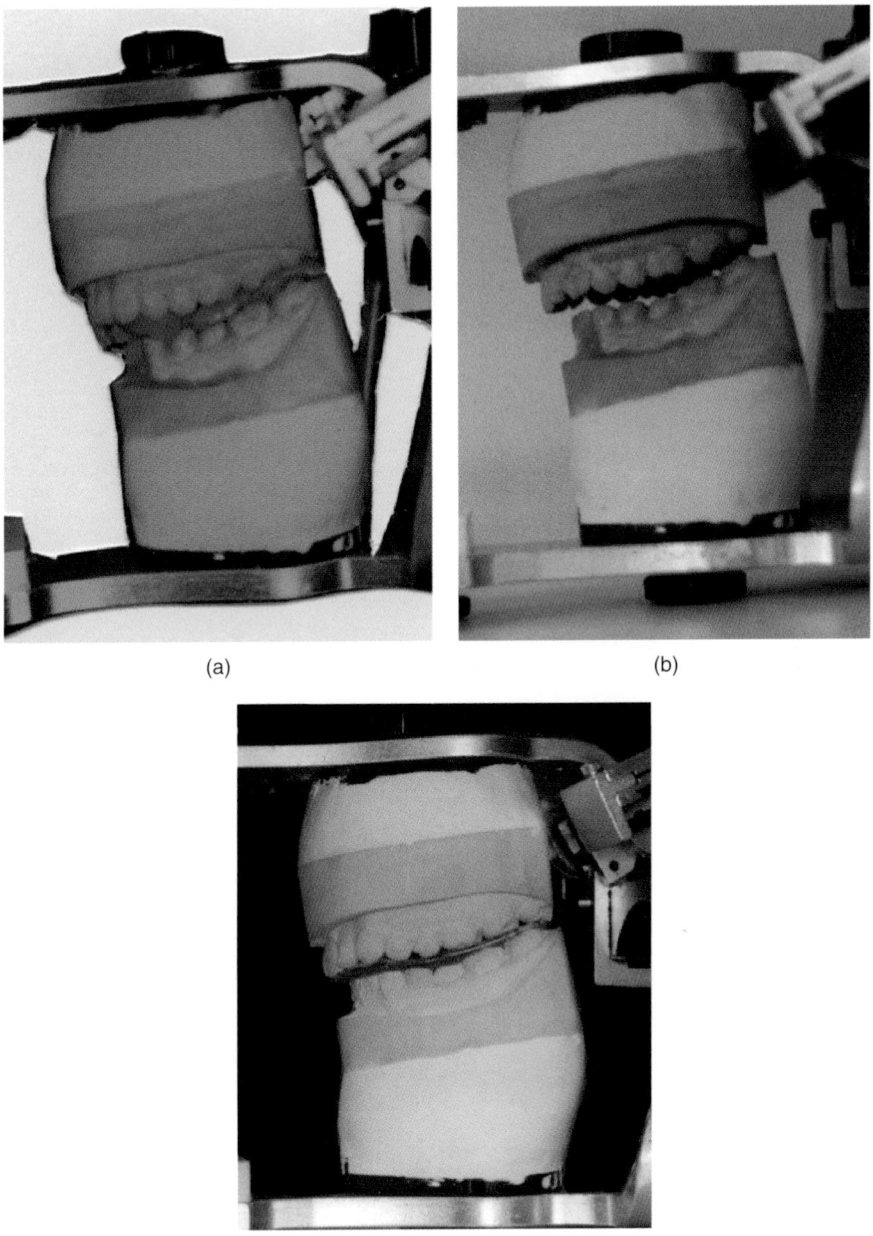

(a)

(b)

(c)

Figure 17.18 Upper and lower models are mounted on a semi-adjustable articulator and a stabilisation splint is constructed in centric relation jaw position, here on the lower model. (a) The models with the bite registration; (b) the models with this registration removed; and (c) the models with the splint inserted. (M. Ziad Al-Ani, Robin J.M. Gray.)

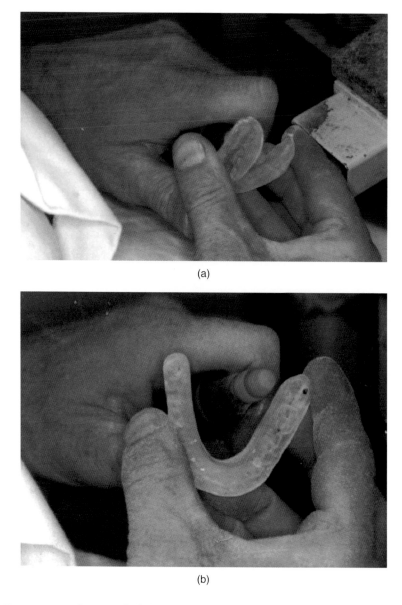

(a)

(b)

Figure 17.19 Adequate relief of undercuts and initial polishing are carried out in the laboratory. (M. Ziad Al-Ani, Robin J.M. Gray.)

Ideal anterior guidance (against the opposing canines and incisors) is developed during lateral excursions, and all posterior interferences, on both the working and non-working sides, are marked and removed.

The easy way to ensure that there are no posterior interferences is to have a steep ramp anteriorly, against which the canines slide. This is unnecessary and undesirable, however, as patients find it easier to move

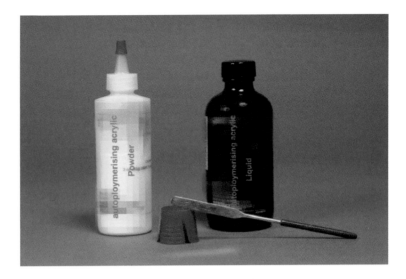

Figure 17.20 Autopolymerising acrylic is used to reline stabilisation splint intraorally at the chairside to provide positive retention. (M. Ziad Al-Ani, Robin J.M. Gray.)

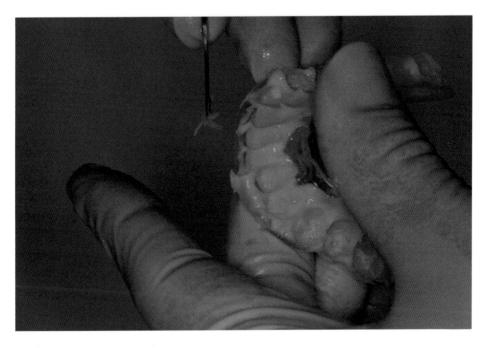

Figure 17.21 The SS was relined with autopolymerising acrylic intraorally at the chairside to provide good and positive retention. The splint must be removed from the mouth before the acrylic has fully set and, when it has set, any excess is removed. (M. Ziad Al-Ani, Robin J.M. Gray.)

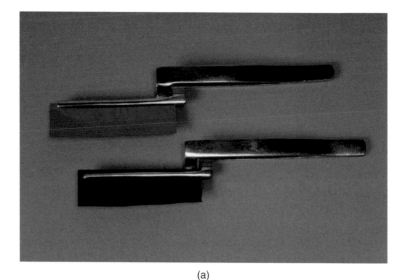

(a)

(b)

Figure 17.22 (a) Thin articulating papers (two different colours) and (b) straight handpiece with grinding stones are used for adjusting the stabilisation splint. (M. Ziad Al-Ani, Robin J.M. Gray.)

laterally on shallow anterior guidance with minimal separation of the posterior teeth.

Once the crossover canine position has been reached, when the lower canine in lateral mandibular excursion has moved lateral to the maxillary canine, the splint is adjusted so that the anterior guidance is transferred to the central incisors, which provide most of the guidance during protrusive movements. As a consequence of wearing the splint, and with the passage of time, muscle relaxation may allow the mandible to adopt a new position. The splint will then need further rebalancing to this

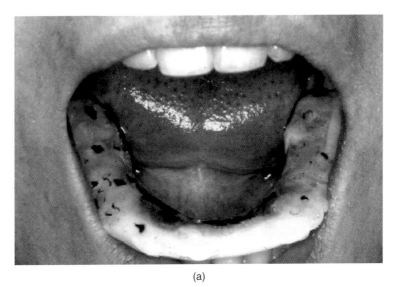

(a)

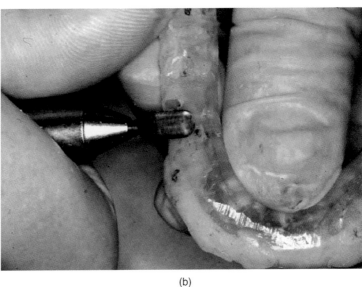

(b)

Figure 17.23 (a) Centric relation stops marked using blue articulating paper; (b) balancing splint by adjusting contacts; (c) development of canine guidance using red articulating paper; (d) canine guidance (red); (e) posterior interferences marked and removed; and (f) balanced splint. (M. Ziad Al-Ani, Robin J.M. Gray.)

new position, until eventually a reproducible centric relation position is established (Figure 17.23).

How do you make an anterior repositioning splint?

Upper and lower models of the patient's dental arches are cast from alginate impressions using Die-stone.

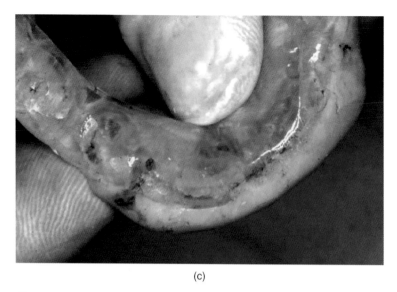

(c)

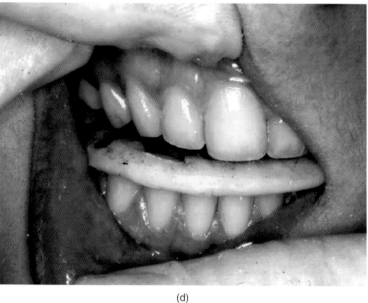

(d)

Figure 17.23 *(Continued)*

For an anterior repositioning splint (ARPS) to be regarded as appropriate treatment, it is important to determine whether the click is eliminated by protrusion of the mandible. At the chairside, the patient is asked to protrude the mandible and then perform a series of opening and closing mouth movements. If the click is eliminated in this protrusive mandibular position, provision of an ARPS is deemed to be suitable treatment (Figure 17.24).

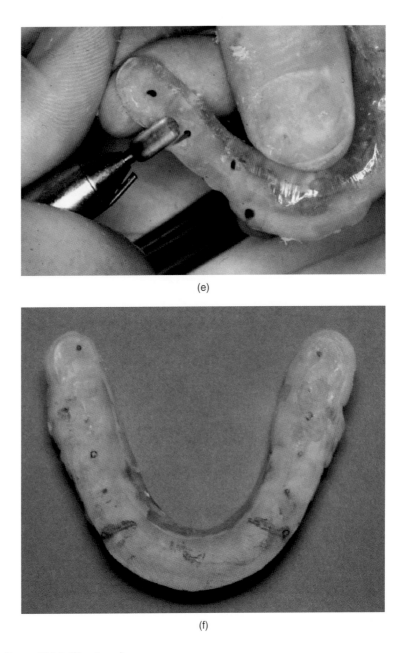

(e)

(f)

Figure 17.23 (*Continued*)

Bite registration

The patient is asked to open the mouth wide and carefully close to a protrusive position, usually in an edge-to-edge incisal relationship to determine whether the click has disappeared. Once this 'click-free' protrusive bite position is achieved, this position is recorded using softened

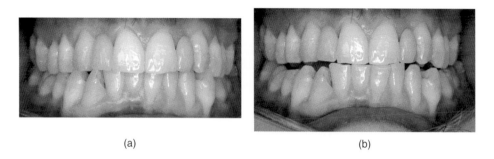

(a)   (b)

Figure 17.24 (a, b) To determine whether the click is eliminated by protrusion of the mandible, the patient is asked to protrude the mandible and then perform a series of opening and closing mouth movements. (M. Ziad Al-Ani, Robin J.M. Gray.)

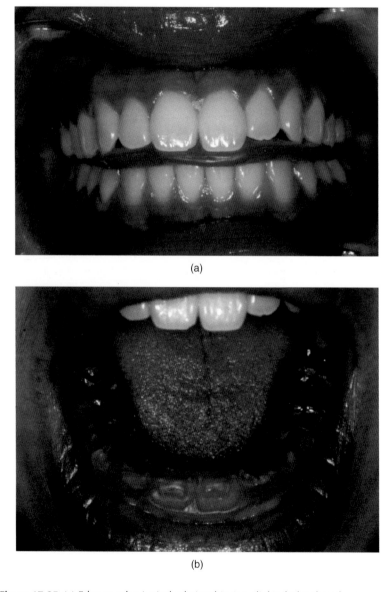

(a)

(b)

Figure 17.25 (a) Edge-to-edge incisal relationship (no click); (b) hardened wax occlusal record can be tested to ensure that the opening and closing cycles are 'click free'. (M. Ziad Al-Ani, Robin J.M. Gray.)

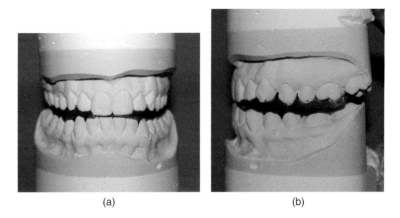

(a)   (b)

Figure 17.26 Upper and lower models with mandible repositioned anteriorly with the wax occlusal record. (M. Ziad Al-Ani, Robin J.M. Gray.)

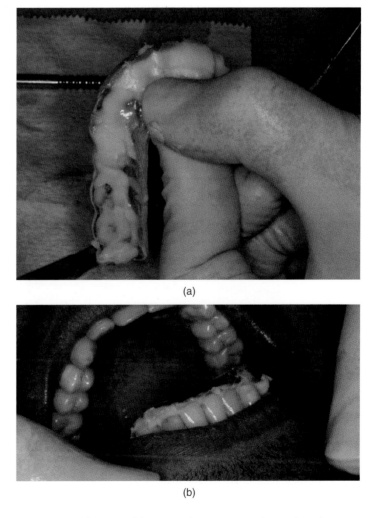

(a)

(b)

Figure 17.27 (a) Application of the autopolymerising acrylic used to reline anterior repositioning splint intraorally at the chairside to provide good and positive retention; (b) the splint placed on to the teeth and fully seated. (M. Ziad Al-Ani, Robin J.M. Gray.)

modelling wax. When the wax has hardened, the click-free position is then checked using the hardened wax as a template (Figures 17.25 and 17.26).

Fitting the ARPS

The splint will be delivered from the laboratory with adequate relief of undercuts to ensure easy seating. The ARPS should be relined with autopolymerising acrylic intraorally at the chairside to provide good and positive retention. While relining, the acrylic is applied to the entire fitting surface of the splint, which is then placed on to the teeth and fully seated. The splint must be removed from the mouth before the acrylic has fully set and, when it has set, any excess is removed using an acrylic trimmer in a straight handpiece. It should then be tried to ensure that it is not too tight but that there is good retention (Figure 17.27).

At the chairside the ARPS is placed in the mouth and checked intraorally by asking the patient to occlude in the new protruded position. This position has been obtained by indentations on the occlusal surface of the splint, into which the patient fits the opposing teeth after protruding the mandible (Figure 17.28).

The operator can confirm the elimination of the click by using the stereo-stethoscope during opening and closing.

No occlusal adjustment should be necessary (Figure 17.29).

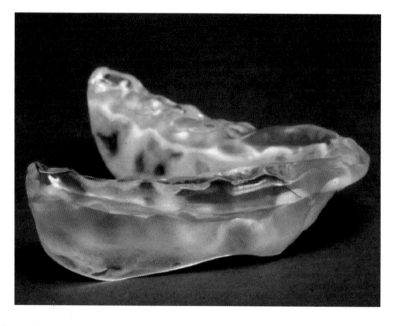

Figure 17.28 Anterior repositioning splint with indentations and ramps to guide the upper teeth into a specific protrusive position. (M. Ziad Al-Ani, Robin J.M. Gray.)

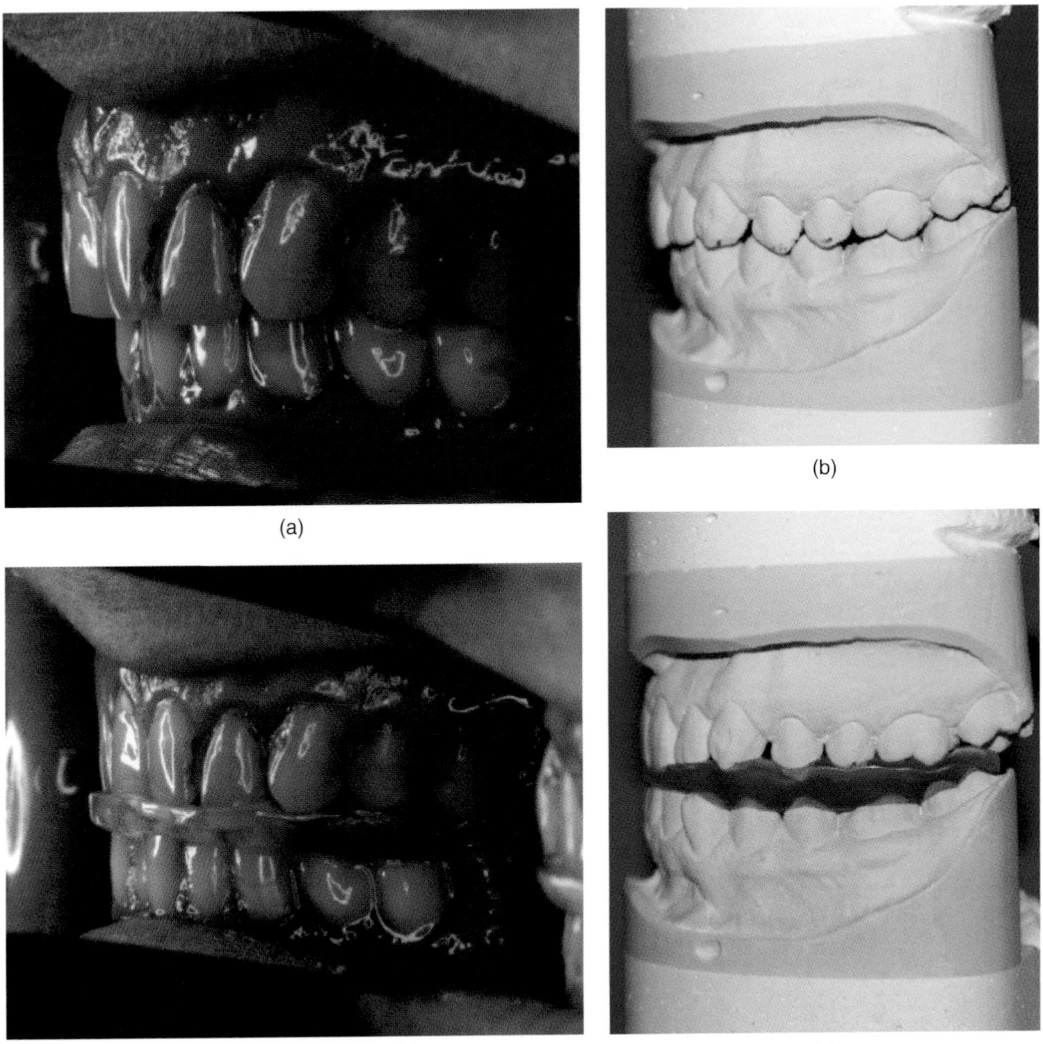

Figure 17.29 (a, b) Teeth in centric occlusion; (c, d) teeth in anterior reposition with splint. (M. Ziad Al-Ani, Robin J.M. Gray.)

Further reading

Galeković, N.H., Fugošić, V., Braut, V., and Ćelić, R. (2017). Reproducibility of centric relation techniques by means of condyle position analysis. *Acta Stomatol Croat* 51: 13–21.

Keshvad, A. and Winstanley, R.B. (2003). Comparison of the replicability of routinely used centric relation registration techniques. *J Prosthodont* 12: 90–101.

Moufti, M.A., Lilico, J.T., and Wassell, R.W. (2007). How to make a well fitting stabilization splint. *Dent Update* 34: 398–400, 402–4, 407–8.

Wilson, P.H. and Banerjee, A. (2004). Recording the retruded contact position: a review of clinical techniques. *Br Dent J* 196: 395–402. quiz 426.

Chapter 18

Bruxism: Current Knowledge of Aetiology and Management

Aetiology of bruxism

In the past, morphological factors such as occlusal discrepancies and the anatomy of the bony structures of the orofacial region have been considered to be the principal aetiological factors for bruxism. The studies have, however, found similar prevalence in sleep bruxism for people with or without occlusal interferences, and sleep bruxism was not reduced by occlusal therapy.

According to the lack of scientific proof for the role of occlusion in the aetiology of bruxism, the morphological theory has been considered to play only a small role, if any.

More recently, the central (pathophysiological and psychological) theory has been postulated by several authors. This suggests that bruxism is associated with the rapid eye movement period of sleep (usually half an hour to an hour before waking). In fact, this view relates bruxism to the autonomic nervous system, that the bruxing mechanism is different from that of chewing and that the teeth play a minor role in the aetiology of bruxism. In other words, the recent view is based on the theory that bruxism appears to be mainly regulated centrally, not peripherally and many literature reviews reveal a tendency to attach less importance to the role of peripheral (e.g., occlusal) factors, and more to centralised ones (e.g., arousal responses, stress, anxiety, temperamental traits).

The most plausible explanation of the aetiopathogenesis of bruxism hypothesises the existence of a multifactorial model in which psychosocial and pathophysiological factors interact with peripheral morphological stimuli.

Several studies have demonstrated a high anxiety trait and increased depressive symptoms as well as an inclination to react with muscle tension and these signs were more evident in bruxists tending to support the central theory. The link between sleep bruxism and psychosocial factors such as emotional stress was supported by the studies reporting elevated levels of urinary catecholamine in patients with sleep bruxism.

However, as the role of psychological factors differs between individuals, it has been suggested that there is a need for more controlled studies in order to confirm or refute this role in the aetiology of bruxism.

Sleep posture has been suggested as an aetiological factor in bruxism. Some studies found that some sleep postures apply lateral forces to the mandible and this was significantly related to the incidence and severity of nocturnal bruxism.

It has been postulated that genetic factors may also play a role as a predisposing factor in bruxism. This theory is based on the fact that monozygotic twins have been demonstrated to have a higher degree of similarity in tooth facet pattern when compared to dizygotic twins. A review of the literature involving DNA analysis, family, and twin studies concluded that sleep bruxism does indeed "run in families" and it appears to be a persistent trait with 35–90% of childhood sleep bruxism will persist into adulthood.

A recent systematic review of published case reports found that there is some evidence that bruxism and jaw pain may be associated with selective serotonin reuptake inhibitors and serotonin–norepinephrine reuptake inhibitors use. The authors of the review suggested that bruxism may develop as an adverse reaction to antidepressant therapy and is most likely to develop within two to three weeks of medication introduction or dose titration. They argued that antidepressant-associated bruxism may be an underreported condition, particularly in the neurology clinic and recommended further prospective trials to help elucidating optimal therapies for this condition.

Study of the aetiology of bruxism is complicated by the existence of diagnostic framing difficulties and, therefore, different controversial opinions have emerged in the literature. It seems, therefore, to be difficult to confirm or refute any of the previously suggested aetiological theories of bruxism. The multifactorial aetiology, appears to be supported by different authors.

Definition of bruxism

Different definitions of bruxism have been described in the literature. In 2012, a written consensus discussion was held among an international group of bruxism experts as to formulate a definition of bruxism and to suggest a grading system for its operationalisation. The expert group defined bruxism as 'a repetitive jaw-muscle activity characterised by clenching or grinding of the teeth and/or by bracing or thrusting of the mandible'.

The old definition of 'diurnal bruxism' refers to habitual parafunction, whilst 'nocturnal bruxism' is a term used to describe tooth grinding, which usually occurs during sleep.

A recent consensus paper suggested that this definition employs 'diurnal' and 'nocturnal' as indicators for the condition's circadian relationships, while 'sleep' and 'awake' are to be preferred for their unbiased nature (some of us sleep during the day and are awake at night).

Bruxism, therefore, has two distinct circadian manifestations: it can occur during sleep (indicated as sleep bruxism) or during wakefulness (indicated as awake bruxism).

'Parafunction' is another term which is suggested to be synonymous with the term bruxism, although the term may be used to describe other habitual behaviours.

Since bruxist activity is mainly performed subconsciously, determining its prevalence of by using questioning alone is therefore unreliable. However, studies by questionnaire have demonstrated that about 15–20% of people are aware of clenching or grinding the teeth. Patients can, however, grind or clench their teeth without producing noise. You must not dismiss the possibility of parafunctional habits just because their sleeping partner has not heard them!

Bruxism and TMD

An awareness of bruxism can be reported but a direct cause and effect relationship is difficult to establish. Mild forms of bruxism rarely have severe consequences for oral structures.

Bruxism can sometimes pose a threat to the integrity of the structures of the masticatory system if the magnitude and direction of the forces exerted exceed the system's adaptive capacity. In extreme cases, however, bruxism can cause tooth structure breakdown, and it has been suggested that this can play a role in the development of a temporomandibular disorder (TMD).

Mild forms of bruxism have rarely any severe consequences for oral structures. In extreme cases, however, bruxism can cause tooth structure breakdown. Moreover, many authors have suggested that it can play a role in the development of a TMD.

It has been suggested that prolonged muscle tension in bruxism leads to aseptic non-serous inflammation in the connective tissue component of the masticatory muscles and a subsequent fatigue and pain similar to that reported by TM dysfunction patients.

In 2016, a paper suggested that until additional studies of the nature proposed above are completed, it is considered premature to consider sleep bruxism more than a behaviour that may lead to harm, but as yet cannot be considered a harmful dysfunction itself (i.e. disorder) or even a risk factor for harmful oral health outcomes.

A systematic review of articles published in the PubMed database over the past decade has been conducted to study bruxism–TMD relationship. It concluded that studies based on more quantitative and specific methods to diagnose bruxism showed a low association with TMD symptoms. Anterior tooth wear was not found to be a major risk factor for TMD.

In light of the available scientific evidence, it is doubtful that bruxism is a direct cause of temporomandibular joint (TMJ) pain and, therefore, treatment strategies focused on controlling bruxism to decrease pain may not be the best solution for patients showing both conditions. Further research is needed into this association bruxism and TMD with higher methodology.

Why bruxism (parafunction) is potentially damaging?

Teeth only come together in ICP for 17.5 minutes a day (500 swallowing contacts) and at other times, the mandible is at rest leaving a gap of a few millimetres between upper and lower teeth. Prolonged heavy contacts (bruxism) are potentially damaging. Furthermore, the amount of pressure paced on teeth during parafunctional habits can range from (2.07 to 20.7 MPa) while bruxing. This, in turn, places significantly more stress on the muscles of mastication.

How much evidence about the efficacy of botulinum toxins on bruxism?

To date, the efficacy of botulinum toxins on bruxism has not been demonstrated. A systematic review of randomised controlled trials and non-randomised studies has been conducted to assess the efficacy of botulinum toxins on bruxism.

One review suggested that botulinum toxin injections can reduce the frequency of bruxism events, decrease bruxism-induced pain levels, and satisfy patients' self-assessment of the effectiveness on bruxism. They found that botulinum toxin injections are equally as effective as nocturnal oral splint for bruxism and botulinum toxin injections at a dosage below 100 U of the masseter or temporalis muscles for otherwise healthy patients are safe. However, only two of the studies – randomised controlled trials – were of high quality and were used in this review, and no research has been performed on the effects of botulinum on sleep quality improvement. The authors concluded that further studies, especially randomised controlled trials of high quality, directed towards the comparison of botulinum toxin injections and oral nocturnal splint, and the effect of botulinum on sleep quality, are urgently needed to explore the advantages of botulinum toxin injections and to promote their wider clinical application.

Some authors used video-polysomnographic records to investigate the effects of intramuscular botulinum toxin type A injection on jaw motor episodes. They compared the effects of injecting this material on jaw motor episodes between the injection sites of the masseter muscle injection only versus injection of both masseter and temporalis muscles. It was found that a single injection of botulinum toxin type A was an effective strategy for controlling sleep bruxism for at least a month as it reduced the intensity rather than the generation of the contraction in jaw-closing muscles. The authors suggested, however, that future investigations on the efficacy and safety in larger samples over a longer follow-up period are needed before establishing management strategies for sleep bruxism with botulinum toxin type A.

Other studies, however, showed that botulinum toxin injections did not change the occurrence but reduced the intensity of contractions for the masseter and temporalis muscles during sleep.

A systematic review of the literature has been conducted to assess the effects of botulinum toxin injections in the management of bruxism and found that despite the paucity of works on the topic, botulinum toxin type A seems to be a possible management option for sleep bruxism, minimising symptoms, and reducing the intensity of muscle contractions. The authors suggested, however, that further studies are necessary especially as far as the treatment indications for bruxism itself is concerned.

A more recent review, compared eleven studies regarding the effectiveness of botulinum toxins on the reduction in the frequency of bruxism events and myofascial pain after injection. The authors of these studies concluded that botulinum toxin could be used as an effective treatment for reducing nocturnal bruxism and myofascial pain in patients with bruxism. They argued, however, that evidence-based research was limited on this topic and more randomised controlled studies are needed to confirm that botulinum toxin is safe and reliable for routine clinical use in bruxism.

Recent findings in animal studies where botulinum toxin was delivered to muscles of mastication show a reduction in bone volume and hypertrophic bone proliferation in and around TMJ. This finding clearly raises concern about botulinum toxin's long-term use and further research is required to prove potential benefits outweigh risks of treatment.

Overall, randomised controlled trials are still very limited in this field and further randomised controlled trials of high quality, directed towards the comparison of botulinum toxin injections and oral splints, and to prove the long-term safety of the material are urgently needed to explore the advantages of botulinum toxin injections and to promote their wider clinical application.

Therefore, Botox is not approved in the United Kingdom for the treatment of bruxism, temporomandibular muscle and joint disorder or for slimming of the lower face.

How can bruxism be managed? 8

Pharmacological, psychological, and dental strategies had been employed to manage sleep bruxism. There is at present, no effective treatment that 'cures' or 'stops' sleep bruxism permanently. A combination of different strategies may be warranted to protect teeth/restorations, reduce bruxism activity, relieve pain and to treat the pathological effects of bruxism on the structures of the masticatory system.

Recent studies suggested that bruxism can best be managed following the so-called 'triple-P' approach: Plates, Pep talk, and Pills. This approach 'reflects the current insight into the aetiology of bruxism, that is considered to be mainly regulated centrally; not peripherally. The approach also stresses that whenever bruxism treatment is indicated, it should be assessed by a multidisciplinary team that includes dentists, psychologists, and medical specialists'.

Further reading

Castrillon, E.E. and Exposto, F.G. (2018). Sleep bruxism and pain. *Dent Clin North Am* 62: 657–663.

Lobbezoo, F. and Naeije, M. (2001). Bruxism is mainly regulated centrally, not peripherally. *J Oral Rehabil* 28: 1085–1091.

Lobbezoo, F., van der Zaag, J., Selms, M.K.A. et al. (2008). Principles for the management of bruxism. *J Oral Rehabil.* 35: 509–523.

Lobbezoo, F., Ahlberg, J., Glaros, A.G. et al. (2013). Bruxism defined and graded: an international consensus. *J Oral Rehabil* 40: 2–4.

Lobbezoo, F., Visscher, C.M., Ahlberg, J., and Manfredini, D. (2014). Bruxism and genetics: a review of the literature. *J Oral Rehabil* 41: 709–714.

Manfredini, D., Bucci, M.B., Sabattini, V.B., and Lobbezoo, F. (2011). Bruxism: overview of current knowledge and suggestions for dental implants planning. *Cranio* 29: 304–312.

Murali, R.V., Rangarajan, P., and Mounissamy, A. (2015). Bruxism: Conceptual discussion and review. *J Pharm Bioallied Sci* 7 (Suppl 1): S265–S270.

Rafferty, K.L., Liu, Z.J., Ye, W. et al. (2012). Botulinum toxin in masticatory muscles: short- and long-term effects on muscle, bone, and craniofacial function in adult rabbits. *Bone* 50: 651–662.

Raphael, K.G., Santiago, V., and Lobbezoo, F. (2016). Is bruxism a disorder or a behaviour? Rethinking the international consensus on defining and grading of bruxism. *J Oral Rehabil* 43: 791–798.

Shim, Y.J., Lee, M.K., Kato, T. et al. (2014). Effects of botulinum toxin on jaw motor events during sleep in sleep bruxism patients: a polysomnographic evaluation. *J Clin Sleep Med* 10: 291–298.

Tinastepe, N., Küçük, B.B., and Oral, K. (2015). Botulinum toxin for the treatment of bruxism. *Cranio* 33: 291–298.

Yap, A.U. and Chua, A.P. (2016). Sleep bruxism: current knowledge and contemporary management. *J Conserv Dent* 19: 383–389.

Evidence-based dentistry

Canales, G.D.T., Câmara-Souza, M., Amaral, C.F. et al. (2017). Is there enough evidence to use botulinum toxin injections for bruxism management? A systematic literature review. *Clin Oral Investigat* 21: s00.

Garrett, A.R. and Hawley, J.S. (2018). SSRI-associated bruxism: a systematic review of published case reports. *Neurol Clin Pract* 8: 135–141.

Joo S, Y., Lee, M.K., Kato, T. et al. (2014). Effects of botulinum toxin on jaw motor events during sleep in sleep bruxism patients: a polysomnographic evaluation. *J Clin Sleep Med* 10: 291–298.

Long, H., Liao, Z., Wang, Y. et al. (2012). Efficacy of botulinum toxins on bruxism: an evidence-based review. *Int Dent J* 62: 1–5.

Manfredini, D. and Lobbezoo, F. (2010). Relationship between bruxism and temporomandibular disorders: a systematic review of literature from 1998 to 2008. *Oral Surg Oral Med Oral Pathol Oral Radiol Endod* 109: e26–e50.

Chapter 19

Splint Therapy for the Management of TMD Patients: An Evidence-Based Discussion

All treatment should be evidence-based. Many common procedures in clinical dentistry are not supported by strong scientific evidence. It is widely accepted that the strongest evidence is found in systematic reviews and randomised controlled clinical trials (RCTs).

The director of The Swedish Council on Technology Assessment in Health Care (SBU) states that 'Any doctor or other professional caregiver who disregards evidence is a charlatan. Only with evidence as your foundation can you take an empathetic, value-oriented and individual approach to your patients'.

Evidence-based studies, however, are difficult to design and implement, and the results are not always easy to interpret and translate into clinical practice. Reviews have suggested a lack of strong evidence for many procedures in dentistry resulting in conflicting opinions.

According to evidence-based dentistry, however, dental practitioners should use the best possible current evidence when making decisions about the treatment of each patient, integrating individual clinical expertise with the best available clinical evidence as well as the patients' wishes and preferences.

Numerous treatments, either on their own or in combination, have been proposed in accordance with various aetiological theories of temporomandibular disorder (TMD). A wide range of pharmacological, occlusal alteration, psychotherapeutic, and physiotherapeutic treatments have also been suggested for the management of TMD, mainly aimed at the reduction of pain and improving the range of movement.

This is possibly the area of most contention in TMD management. Several treatments have been proposed which are not evidence- or science-based and when the literature is critically evaluated, it is obvious they have little rationale. It is not sufficient to argue that if a treatment modality is published in a journal, which may not be subject to peer

Temporomandibular Disorders: A Problem-Based Approach, Second Edition. M. Ziad Al-Ani and Robin J.M. Gray.
© 2021 M. Ziad Al-Ani and Robin J.M. Gray. Published 2021 by John Wiley & Sons Ltd.
Companion Website: www.wiley.com/go/al-ani/temporomandibular-disorders-2e

review, be un-refereed, or is accessible through the Internet, then it is validated. The dentist has a responsibility only to prescribe treatment for patients that has a proven therapeutic value and ignorance of currently accepted views of what a reasonable body of dentists would do is not an excuse.

The management of patients with temporomandibular disorders is controversial and attracts suggestions from widely differing viewpoints. Such patients are, after all, suffering from a common musculoskeletal disorder like many others. The use of occlusal splints is, however, commonly accepted, and occlusal splint therapy should be regarded as one of the readily accessible treatments for TMD available to general dental practitioners.

The following have all been recommended as theories for 'successful' mechanisms of treatment:

- The temporary elimination of occlusal interferences
- A placebo effect
- A temporomandibular joint/condylar repositioning effect
- An increased vertical dimension
- Reduced activity in the muscles of mastication secondary to a change in reflex patterns
- An increased stability between the maxilla and mandible.

Stabilisation splint (SS) 7

A number of clinical studies have specifically evaluated the treatment of myofascial pain by stabilisation splint (SS) therapy and clinical success has been reported. When properly adjusted (Figure 19.1a,b), the SS delivers a good method of providing centric relation occlusion (the position of the jaw relative to the skull when the muscles are at their most relaxed and least strained position), eliminating posterior interferences, providing anterior guidance on anterior teeth, reducing neuromuscular activity, and obtaining stable occlusal relationships with uniform tooth contacts throughout the dental arch.

A high clinical success rate of SS therapy in reducing signs and symptoms of myofascial pain has been reported.

It has been demonstrated, by the use of electromyography (EMG) studies, that the use of an SS leads to reduced activity of the masticatory muscles, and many authors reported a reduction in EMG activity of both the anterior temporalis and the masseter muscles in patients with myofascial pain after wearing an SS at night, indicating that nocturnal masticatory muscle activity, both in bruxism and clenching, can be reduced by splint usage.

Other studies showed a significant improvement in myofascial pain signs and symptoms in patients who used an SS in three different patterns (24 hours/day, only during the day, and only at night). It has been demonstrated that patients with myofascial pain only need to wear the splint

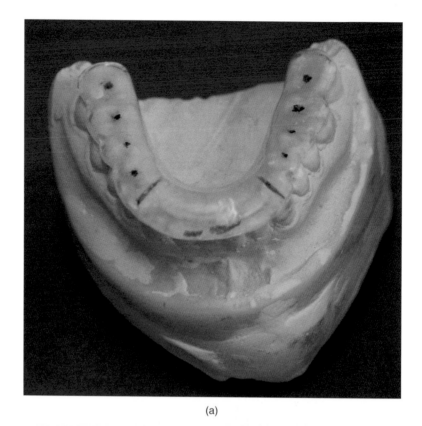

(a)

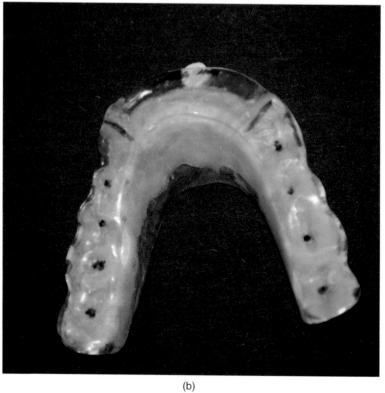

(b)

Figure 19.1 Properly adjusted stabilisation splint. (M. Ziad Al-Ani, Robin J.M. Gray.)

at night, as no greater improvement was found with increased usage. In a subsequent study, the same authors conducted a long-term follow-up of those myofascial pain patients successfully treated with the SS. They demonstrated that 88%, who improved, reported maintenance of their improvement at three-year follow-up.

It was concluded that SS is a successful long-term treatment for myofascial pain and that there is no need, in the overwhelming majority of patients, for 'second phase' permanent alteration of the patient's occlusion either by means of orthodontic treatment or by advanced restorative treatment.

Some studies showed that, after 12 months of use, SS was found still to have been effective in the alleviation of signs and symptoms in TMD patients.

Using computerised EMG before and after using an SS in 22 TMD patients, it was reported that the SS reduced the electrical activity of both masseter and anterior temporalis muscles.

Moreover, using high-resolution gray-scale ultrasonography, it has been demonstrated that the use of an SS was effective in the reduction of muscle bulk in TMD patients. A significant decrease in the cross-sectional dimensions of the masseter muscle in TMD patients after SS usage was also shown.

Although the mechanisms of action of splints are not fully understood, some recent studies suggested that an increased calcitonin gene related peptide was found in TMD patients treated with an occlusal splint. This neuropeptide is thought to play a significant role in decreasing activity muscles responsible for myofascial pain.

Some authors, however, proposed that splints decrease pain by preventing tooth contact and reducing muscle tension.

A Cochrane systematic review compared SS therapy to acupuncture, bite plates, biofeedback/stress management, visual feedback, relaxation, jaw exercises, non-occluding appliance, and minimal/no treatment. The authors concluded that there was no evidence of a statistically significant difference in the effectiveness of SS therapy in reducing symptoms in patients with myofascial pain compared with other active treatments. The authors stated that there is weak evidence to suggest that the use of SS for the treatment of myofascial pain may be beneficial for reducing pain severity, at rest and on palpation, when compared to no treatment.

This review suggests the need for further, well conducted RCTs that pay attention to method of allocation, outcome assessment, large sample size, and enough duration of follow-up. A standardisation of the outcomes of the treatment of myofascial pain should be established in the RCTs.

SS therapy, therefore, appears to have a place in the management of some TMD symptoms but well-conducted RCTs are needed to clarify the effectiveness of SS therapy for patients with myofascial pain. Trials should pay attention to the generation of the randomization sequence, method of allocation, blind outcome assessment, sample size, and duration of follow-up. Clear inclusion/exclusion criteria may help identify whether or not the patients entering a study had myofascial pain or a different diagnosis of temporomandibular disorder.

A standardization of the outcomes used to assess the treatment of myofascial pain should be established in the RCTs.

A recent meta-analysis of short- and long-term effects of SS in TMD patients found that SS presented short-term benefit for patients with TMDs. In long-term follow-up, however, the effect is equalised with other therapeutic modalities. The authors of this review suggested that further studies based on appropriate use of standardised criteria for patient recruitment and outcomes under assessment are needed to better define SS effect persistence in long term.

A single-blinded, randomised clinical trial investigated the therapeutic effects of laser therapy and of an occlusal SS for reducing pain and dysfunction and improving the quality of sleep in patients with TMDs and fibromyalgia syndrome (FMS). The authors concluded that laser therapy or an occlusal SS can be an alternative therapeutic treatment for reducing pain symptoms and the clicking sound for TMDs in patients with FMS.

A recent meta-analysis of randomised controlled trials suggested that the additional use of a hard SS with counselling therapy provides minimal advantage over the use of counselling therapy alone and the authors claimed that starting with low-cost counselling therapy is highly recommended before using a combination of counselling therapy and a hard SS.

Moreover, it has been demonstrated in the same review that the hard SS alone is an effective treatment in reducing signs and symptoms of myogenous TMDs when compared to no treatment (untreated control subjects) or treatment with non-occluding splints. The RCTs involved, however, were of low quality evidence.

Are occlusal splints effective for treating sleep bruxism?

A Cochrane systematic review concluded that there is not sufficient evidence to state that the occlusal splint is effective for treating sleep bruxism. Indication of its use is questionable with regard to sleep outcomes, but it may be that there is some benefit with regard to tooth wear.

This systematic review suggests the need for further investigation in more controlled RCTs that pay attention to method of allocation, outcome assessment, large sample size, and sufficient duration of follow-up. The study design must be parallel, in order to eliminate the bias provided by studies of cross-over type. A standardisation of the outcomes of the treatment of sleep bruxism should be established in the RCTs.

Anterior repositioning splint (ARPS)   7

The anterior repositioning splint (ARPS) is a full coverage splint constructed for the lower arch, which guides the mandible downwards and forwards into a protrusive position to correct a disccondyle incoordination.

Some studies demonstrated that 86% of patients who used an ARPS for 24 hours a day found this splint to be moderately to highly successful at reducing or eliminating temporomandibular joint (TMJ) clicking.

Also, a randomised controlled trial compared patients with disc displacement with reduction (DDwR) wearing an ARPS either during the day, or at night, or all the time. They found that 88% of patients who wore the splint on a 24-hour per day regime had a statistically significant reduction in clicking over a three-month period when compared with the other two groups. It was concluded that the ARPS is an appropriate treatment for patients suffering from DDwR, provided that it is used for 24 hours a day throughout the treatment period. Also, some authors conducted a long-term follow-up of patients with DDwR successfully treated by ARPS. They found that 90% of these patients reported maintenance of their improvement after three years. They concluded that the ARPS is successful for the management of DDwR without the need to resort to any form of permanent second phase treatment.

These findings have been substantiated by other authors. In a study of 160 patients with DDwR treated with an ARPS, a success rate of 89.4% was reported. They demonstrated that the average time for the initial remission of symptoms was 21 days, while the average time for the final remission of symptoms was 130 days.

Using magnetic resonance imaging (MRI), some authors evaluated disc repositioning after the insertion of an ARPS and showed that 70% of anteriorly displaced discs were 'recaptured' by the insertion of the appliance.

MRI and clinical findings have been used to assess factors which influenced the success of disc recapture by the insertion of the ARPS. It was demonstrated that joints with DDwR had successful disc recapture after splint therapy. However, joints exhibiting disc displacement without reduction, or with the presence of inflammatory conditions, with changed disc morphology and extensive disc displacement were negative factors that affected the success.

Other studies demonstrated that MRI showed recapture of the disc in 15 out of 18 DDwR cases. There was no recapture in disc displacement without reduction joints, nor in joints with degenerative changes.

A recent report has showed that 72 juvenile patients with 91 joints (DDwR) were treated with ARPS therapy had a success rate was 92.31% at the end of treatment and 72.53% after 12 months.

It was concluded that ARPS used as a functional appliance could help re-establish a normal disc-condylar relationship. However, a larger sample with longer follow-up are also required to fully determine the long-term efficacy of ARPS.

Another recent study evaluated the efficacy of ARPS for the treatment of DDwR showed a significant reduction of pain in the area of the temporomandibular joints. They assumed that this treatment option is effective upon painful DDwR.

The study concluded that the anterior repositioning splint is an efficient tool in decreasing pain related to DDwR.

Another study explored the effects of ARPS on disc–condyle angles and disc/condyle positions using MRI metric analysis. Upon ARPS insertion, all TMJs with anterior disc displacement with reduction (ADDwR) were found to achieve ideal spatial disc–condyle relationships. The latter was achieved by significant forward and downward movement of the condyles and concurrent backward movement of the discs. The stability of this relationship could not be maintained in the majority of TMJs upon ARPS removal, six months after splint treatment. Normal disc–condyle relationships were observed in only 40–60% of joints with ADDwR. The majority of condyles returned to their posterior pre-treatment positions while the discs generally moved anteriorly again. These findings provided new insights into the short-term and longer term effectiveness of ARPS.

Do occlusal contacts change following splint therapy?

Some authors compared the mean number of occlusal contacts before and after occlusal appliance therapy in three TMD groups and one control group. Only patients with a clinically successful treatment outcome were considered in the statistical analysis. No significant change in the pre- and post-treatment mean number of occlusal contacts between first and final reviews was seen in myofascial pain or bruxism groups, following splint therapy.

However, a statistically significant change in the number of occlusal contacts was reported in the DDwR group, managed with ARPS. In this group, three months after weaning off the splint, when the disc appeared to be returned to position, the mean number of contacts was increased significantly and approached the mean of the other groups (Table 19.1). When the disc is out of position, therefore, the number of occlusal contacts appears to be reduced. It would appear to be sound advice not to make permanent and irreversible adjustment to the occlusion, or undertake extensive restorative treatment in the presence of acute disc displacement as, when the disc repositions, occlusal contacts appear inevitably to exhibit change.

Table 19.1 The mean total number of occlusal contacts at first and third reviews for the myofascial pain group, bruxism group and disc displacement with reduction group.

Group	Number of patients	Mean number of occlusal contacts at 1st review	Mean number of occlusal contacts at 3rd review (after weaning off)
Myofascial pain	68	35.19	34.79
Bruxism	77	37.04	36.37
DDwR	63	25.28	34.47

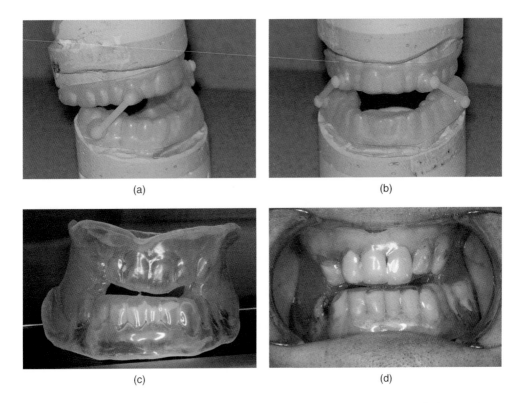

(a)

(b)

(c)

(d)

Figure 19.2 (a–d) Custom made mandibular advancement/snoring appliances. (M. Ziad Al-Ani, Robin J.M. Gray.)

Mandibular advancement/snoring appliances

Dentists are being approached by patients and commercial companies with increasing frequency to provide appliances for those who suffer with anti-social snoring. Several designs are proposed, some are custom made but many are not (Figure 19.2a–d). The practitioner should be wary of prescribing non-custom made appliances.

As a profession, we warn patients away from 'boil and bite' mouthguards. They do not fit well, they are not made to the dentist's prescription and they do not distribute forces evenly, rendering their benefit dubious.

The same is true of other pre-formed occlusal appliances. The provision of an 'anti-snoring appliance' requires careful collaboration between dentist and technician to determine whether the articulatory system will support such a splint. If there is any doubt about the periodontal status this should be addressed before suggesting treatment.

Considerable forces are transmitted to the teeth and supporting structures by wearing these, and it is the dentist's responsibility to ensure that exemplary oral hygiene, bone support, and periodontal condition exist otherwise direct damage to the tissues can result.

The degree of mandibular protrusion should be carefully monitored. Too little, and the appliance will not work. Too much and the appliance can have a detrimental effect on the teeth, periodontium, and TMJs and mandibular muscles leading to clinical damage.

Pre-formed anti-snoring appliances are inappropriate when custom made, readily adjustable ones are available.

Partial coverage pre-formed anti-snoring appliances are unjustifiable. Some are packaged with questionnaires for the dentist and patient to complete including questions about 'major life events, drug abuse, and somatisation'. To the majority of snorers (and dentists) such questions are irrelevant and often inappropriate.

Patients may have sought recourse to sleep clinics and will have had sleep apnoea investigation.

In the face of this, the dentist has the responsibility to critically evaluate such dental treatments before suggesting them to patients and thereby endorsing their use.

In general terms, this applies not only to suggested appliance use but also to courses which promote a series of 'quick fix' appliances and courses which have the objective of covering 'all you need to know' about a topic in a day.

The dentist must be aware of and be able to freely discuss the success rate of such treatments and, very importantly, other alternatives. It must be explained to the patient pre-treatment that there are limitations and that there is no guarantee of success in all cases.

Further Reading

Al-Ani, Z., Davies, S., Sloan, P., and Gray, R. (2008). Change in the number of occlusal contacts following splint therapy in patients with a temporomandibular disorder (TMD). *Eur J Prosthodont Restor Dent* 16: 98–103.

Bertram, S., Rudisch, A., Bonder, G., and Emshoff, R. (2002). Effect of stabilistaion splint type splint on the asymmetry of masseter muscle sites during maximal clenching. *J Oral Rehabil* 29: 447–451.

Carlsson, G.E. (2010). Some dogmas related to prosthodontics, temporomandibular disorders and occlusion. *Acta Odontol Scand* 68: 313–322.

Chen, H.M., Liu, M.Q., Yap, A.U., and Fu, K.Y. (2017). Physiological effects of anterior repositioning splint on temporomandibular joint disc displacement: a quantitative analysis. *J Oral Rehabil* 44: 664–672.

Clark, G.T. (1984). A critical evaluation of orthopedic interocclusal appliance therapy. Design, theory, and overall effectiveness. *J Am Dent Assoc* 108: 359–365.

Clark, G.T. (1986). The TMJ repositioning appliance: a technique for construction, insertion, and adjustment. *J Craniomandib Pract* 4: 37--46.

Davies, S.J. and Gray, R.J.M. (1997). The pattern of splint usage in the managament of two common temporomandibular disorders. Part I: the anterior repositioning splint in the treatment of disc displacement with reduction. *Br Dent J* 183: 199–203.

Davies, S.J. and Gray, R.J.M. (1997). The pattern of splint usage in the management of two common temporomandibular disorders. Part II: the stabilisation splint in the treatment of pain dysfunction syndrome. *Br Dent J* 183: 247–251.

Davies, S.J. and Gray, R.J.M. (1997). The pattern of splint usage in the management of two common temporomandibular disorders. Part III: long-term follow-up in an assessment of splint therapy in the management of disc displacement with reduction and pain dysfunction syndrome. *Br Dent J* 183: 279–283.

Eberhard, D., Bantleon, H., and Steger, W. (2002). The efficacy of anterior repositioning splint therapy studied by magnetic resonance imaging. *Eur J Orthod* 24: 343–352.

Ekberg, E. and Nilner, M. (2002). A 6- and 12-month follow-up of appliance therapy in TMD patients: a follow-up of a controlled trial. *Int J Prosthodont* 15: 564–570.

Emshoff, R. and Bertram, S. (1998). The short-term effect of stabilisation-type splints on local cross- sectional dimensions of muscles of the head and neck. *J Prosthet Dent* 80: 457–461.

Gray, R.J., Davies, S.J., and Quayle, A.A. (1994). A clinical approach to temporomandibular disorders. 6 splint therapy. *Br Dent J* 177: 135–142.

Glaros, A.G., Owais, Z., and Lausten, L. (2007). Reduction in parafunctional activity: a potential mechanism for the effectiveness of splint therapy. *J Oral Rehabil* 34: 97–104.

Grant, A.D., Tam, C.W., Lazar, Z. et al. (2004). The calcitonin gene-related peptide (CGRP) receptor antagonist BIBN4096BS blocks CGRP and adrenomedullin vasoactive responses in the microvasculature. *Br J Pharmacol* 142: 1091–1098.

Hiyama, S., Ono, T., ishiwata, Y. et al. (2003). First night effect of an interocclusal appliance on nocturnal masticatory muscle activity. *J Oral Rehabil* 30: 139––145.

Kurita, H., Kurashina, K., and Kotani, A. (1997). Clinical effect of full coverage occlusal splint therapy for specific temporomandibular disorder conditions and symptoms. *J Prosthet Dent* 78: 506–510.

Kurita, H., Kurashina, K., Ohtsuka, A., and Kotani, A. (1998). Change of position of the temporomandibular joint disk with insertion of a disk-repositioning appliance. *Oral Surg Oral Med Oral Pathol Oral Radiol Endod* 85: 142–145.

Kurita, H., Ohtsuka, A., Kurashina, K., and Kopp, S. (2001). A study of factors for successful splint capture of anteriorly displaced temporomandibular joint disc with disc repositioning appliance. *J Oral Rehabil* 28: 651–657.

Landulpho, A.B., WA, E.S., FA, E.S., and Vitti, M. (2004). Electromyographic evaluation of masseter and anterior temporalis muscles in patients with temporomandibular disorders following interocclusal appliance treatment. *J Oral Rehabil* 31: 95––98.

Ma, Z., Xie, Q., Yang, C. et al. (2019). Can anterior repositioning splint effectively treat temporomandibular joint disc displacement? *Sci Rep* 9: 1–8.

Naeije, M. and Hansson, T. (1991). Short-term effect of the stabilisation appliance on masticatory muscle activity in myogenous craniomandibular disorder patients. *J Craniomandib Disord* 5: 245–250.

Niemelä, K., Korpela, M., Raustia, A. et al. (2012). Efficacy of stabilisation splint treatment on temporomandibular disorders. *J Oral Rehabil* 39: 799–804.

Pihut, M., Gorecka, M., Ceranowicz, P., and Wieckiewicz, M. (2018). The efficiency of anterior repositioning splints in the management of pain related to temporomandibular joint disc displacement with reduction. *Pain Res Manag*: 1–6.

Seligman, D.A. and Pullinger, A.G. (1991). The role of functional occlusal relationships in temporomandibular disorders: a review. *J Craniomandibular Disord: Facial Oral Pain* 5: 265–279.

Williamson, E.H. and Rosenzweig, B.J. (1998). The treatment of temporo-mandibular disorders through repositioning splint therapy: a follow-up study. *Cranio* 16: 222–225.

Evidence-based Dentistry

Al-Ani, Z., Gray, R.J., Davies, S.J. et al. (2005). Stabilization splint therapy for the treatment of temporomandibular myofascial pain: a systematic review. *J Dent Educ* 69: 1242–1250.

Al-Moraissi, E.A., Farea, R., Qasem, K.A. et al. (2020). Effectiveness of occlusal splint therapy in the management of temporomandibular disorders: network meta-analysis of randomised controlled trials [published online ahead of print, 2020 Jan 22]. *Int J Oral Maxillofac Surg* S0901-5027 (20): 30004–30007.

Kuzmanovic Pficer, J., Dodic, S., Lazic, V. et al. (2017). Occlusal stabilization splint for patients with temporomandibular disorders: Meta-analysis of short and long term effects. *PLoS One* 12: e0171296.

Macedo, C.R., Silva, A.B., Machado, M.A. et al. (2007). Occlusal splints for treating sleep bruxism (tooth grinding). *Cochrane Database Syst Rev* 4: CD005514.

Molina-Torres, G., Rodríguez-Archilla, A., Matarán-Peñarrocha, G. et al. (2016). Laser therapy and occlusal stabilization splint for temporomandibular disorders in patients with fibromyalgia syndrome: a randomized, Clinical Trial. *Altern Ther Health Med* 22: 23–31.

Nitecka-Buchta, A., Marek, B., and Baron, S. (2014). CGRP plasma level changes in patients with temporomandibular disorders treated with occlusal splints – a randomised clinical trial. *Endokrynol Polska* 65: 217–223.

Zhang, C., Wu, J.Y., Deng, D.L. et al. (2016). Efficacy of splint therapy for the management of temporomandibular disorders: a meta-analysis. *Oncotarget* 7: 84043–84053.

Chapter 20

Patient Information

This chapter contains some examples of patient information leaflets with information that you might like to give to your patients when appropriate.

Stabilisation splint 7

- This splint aims to provide comfortable contact between your opposing teeth and the surface of the splint. This might be to help your jaw muscles relax, to encourage you to stop grinding or clenching your teeth, or to 'balance' your bite.
- Usually, you will need to wear this splint only at night, but please follow the advice of the clinician who is looking after you.
- We find that after successful splint therapy most people can be 'weaned' off their splint and we will advise you about this on an individual basis.
- When you are not wearing your splint remember to keep it in a damp tissue or store it in water.
- Clean your splint with toothpaste and a toothbrush. You can soak it in a dilute solution of Milton for a few hours once a week if necessary. Do not use anything hot to clean it (i.e. boiling water).
- Stop wearing your splint if any of it breaks off and inform us at your next appointment. If you carry on wearing it your teeth could move position.
- We need to review your progress at regular intervals, and also adjust the splint as needed. *Please remember to bring the splint with you each time that you visit.*

Temporomandibular Disorders: A Problem-Based Approach, Second Edition. M. Ziad Al-Ani and Robin J.M. Gray.
© 2021 M. Ziad Al-Ani and Robin J.M. Gray. Published 2021 by John Wiley & Sons Ltd.
Companion Website: www.wiley.com/go/al-ani/temporomandibular-disorders-2e

Anterior repositioning splint 7

- This splint aims to maintain your jaw in a particular position in which there is no click when you open and close your mouth.
- You must wear your splint 24 hours a day, including when eating.
- If your jaw should lock (i.e. you cannot open your mouth very wide) leave the splint out until your next appointment.
- Remove your splint only to clean your teeth and the splint. While the splint is out, your mouth opening should be restricted to avoid causing the click.
- Please try to adhere strictly to a soft diet during the period of splint therapy.
- We will need to review your progress at regular intervals.
- If any of the splint breaks off you should stop wearing it immediately and inform us at your next appointment. If you carry on wearing it your teeth could move position.
- After becoming symptom free, (normally after 12 weeks of splint therapy), you will then be advised about how to wean off splint therapy slowly. **Do not do this on your own.** Your clinician will advise you on the best regimen for you. A common regimen is as follows:

1. Leave the splint out for 1 hour in the morning and 1 hour in the evening for 3–4 days until you get used to being without it.
2. Gradually increase these periods (2, then 3 hours at a time) until your splint is only worn at night. This should take three to four weeks. You might find it more comfortable, at first, to continue wearing the splint when eating because you will initially be aware of a gap between your back teeth. Your bite will return to normal as your jaw goes back to the pre-treatment position.
3. Progressively reduce night-time wear by one night a week, but alternating the nights as far as possible.
4. If you feel that the click might be about to return, go back to wearing the splint for a few days or nights. You will never do any harm by doing this.
5. If you later want to use the splint again and it has dried out, rehydrate it by soaking it in water for 24 hours before trying it. If you feel that it does not fit comfortably then contact your clinician.

Use and care of occlusal bite splint 7

The occlusal bite splint you have received should help to reduce tension in the jaw muscles, decrease painful symptoms, protect the teeth, and/or maintain your jaw in a particular position. The following is a list of information and helpful hints concerning your splint.

The splint should be worn regularly as instructed.

Saliva flow often increases during the first two weeks of wearing the splint. This is normal. Each time the splint is placed over your teeth, it might feel tight for a few minutes. This is normal.

Each time the splint is removed from your mouth, your 'bite' may feel different for several minutes. This is normal.

You may find it difficult to pronounce certain words when the splint is first worn. After a few days, speech will usually return to almost normal.

When the splint is not worn, it should be kept moist. Either place it in water or wrap it in a wet tissue.

Regular check-ups should be made to check the adjustment and fit of your splint. If no ongoing appointments are made, do not wear your splint more than four to six months without having it checked.

Please remember to bring the splint with you each time you attend.

Your splint should be kept clean just as your teeth should. Bad breath and/or a bad taste may result from neglect of your oral hygiene.

Brush your splint gently with a toothbrush and toothpaste.

Try not to bite or clench on the splint. It is intended to help your jaw muscles relax, not exercise.

Table 20.1 lists of foods that are advised and not advised for patients with a temporomandibular disorder (TMD).

Table 20.1 Diet for patients with temporomandibular disorders.

Advised	Not advised
Bread: brown or white bread (crusts removed) and soft rolls	**Bread:** avoid baguettes, bagels, hard rolls
Desserts: all soft puddings	
Dairy foods and eggs: cottage cheese, milk, ice cream	
Fish: any cooked fish	
Fruits: any canned or stewed fruit. Melon, bananas, apples, etc., but cut into thin slices	**Fruits:** avoid whole apples or other hard fruits
Liquids: all beverages; fortified 'liquid meals' are recommended	
Meats: any easily chewed meat such as mince, chicken	**Meats:** avoid steak or any meat that requires excessive chewing
Miscellaneous: any of the variety of nourishing mixtures that can be mixed in a blender (milk shakes, fruit, or vegetable blends)	**Miscellaneous:** no hard or chewy sweets, no gum
Pasta: any cooked pasta	
Potatoes: mashed, baked, or boiled	
Soups: any type of soup	
Vegetables: any cooked fresh frozen or canned vegetables	**Vegetables:** avoid raw vegetables, e.g. carrots, and corn on the cob

General advice for patients with a TMD

1. Cut all food into small bite-size pieces. DO NOT open your mouth any wider than necessary.
2. DO NOT eat hard crusts of bread, tough meat, raw vegetables, chewing gum or anything that requires prolonged chewing.
3. DO NOT bite any food with your front teeth, especially with your mouth open wide (i.e. bite into an apple).
4. When the pain is acute, hot and cold compresses can be used, such as frozen peas for a minute wrapped up in a towel followed by a hot water bottle for two to three minutes, repeating this cycle two or three times (Figure 20.1a,b).
5. Use an anti-inflammatory gel massaged in front of the ear, over the joint. These contain ibuprofen absorbed through the soft tissue and some products also contain levomenthol, which stimulates blood flow.
6. Rest your jaw as much as possible.
7. Once your pain has resolved, an exercise programme might be used, but undertake this ONLY upon the direct advice of your clinician.
8. Do not keep trying to stretch your mouth widely if you feel that your movement is 'tight' or restricted.
9. If your jaw feels locked do NOT try to force it open.

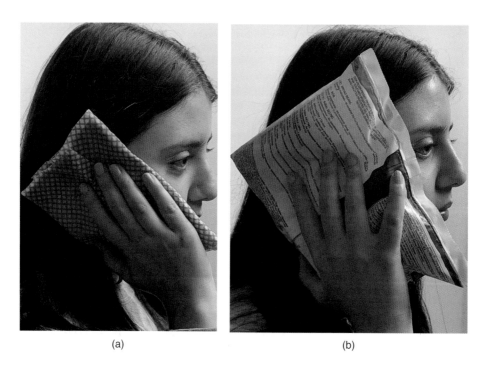

(a)   (b)

Figure 20.1 (a, b) Hot and cold compresses can be used to treat acute pain. (M. Ziad Al-Ani, Robin J.M. Gray).

Exercise programme for patients with TMD

Only do this on the advice of your clinician.

Vertical movement

Place your hand under your chin. Open your mouth to half maximum. Try to close your mouth with your hand but forcibly resist this movement with your jaw. Hold for 10 seconds. Relax and repeat five times.

Lateral movement

- Place your hand on the side of your chin, opposite the affected side. Move your jaw towards your hand. Try to push your jaw back to the midline with your hand but forcibly resist this movement with your jaw. Hold for 10 seconds. Relax and repeat five times.
- Stand in front of a mirror and open and close your mouth to the maximum comfortable range. If your jaw moves to one side, then place your hands on each side of your jaw and apply pressure as appropriate to encourage your lower jaw to open straight. Repeat five times.
- With your mouth slightly open, put your tongue to the outside of your upper teeth on the opposite side to the affected joint. Hold this position for 10 seconds. Relax and repeat five times.

Protrusive movement

Hold a tongue spatula or any other safe flat object, such as a spoon handle, at a 45° angle downwards between your upper and lower teeth with them slightly parted. Push your lower jaw forwards to your maximum along the spatula/handle. Make sure that your lower jaw moves in a straight pathway and does not deviate to one side or another. Hold for 10 seconds. Relax and repeat five times (Figure 20.2a,b).

Perform each exercise in the morning and at night. Morning is important. Do each exercise for about a minute and then gradually build up in time. Operate out of your 'comfort zone' but not to the extent that you cause pain. Your jaw movement has been restricted and will take time to improve.

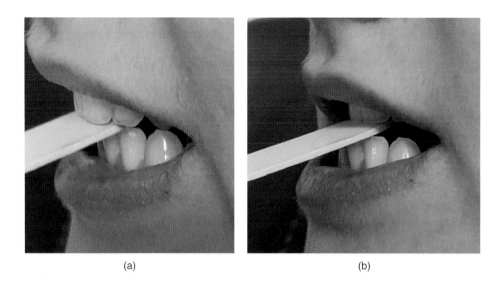

(a)   (b)

Figure 20.2 Protrusive movement using tongue spatula held at 45-degree angle between upper and lower teeth. (M. Ziad Al-Ani, Robin J.M. Gray.)

Appendix I
Flowcharts

Temporomandibular Disorders: A Problem-Based Approach, Second Edition. M. Ziad Al-Ani and Robin J.M. Gray.
© 2021 M. Ziad Al-Ani and Robin J.M. Gray. Published 2021 by John Wiley & Sons Ltd.
Companion Website: www.wiley.com/go/al-ani/temporomandibular-disorders-2e

Patient
Date

1. TMJ Examination
   (Yes = √)

  A. Tenderness on palpation   R   L
    (a) Lateral
    (b) Intra-auricular

  B. Joint sounds   R   L
    Click   Early   Mid   Late
    Opening   Closing
    Painful   Painless
    Crepitus

  C. Range of motion (mm):   maximum   pain-free
    Vertical
    Lateral   R: L:

  D. Pathway of Opening:
    Straight

                               R   L
    Lasting deviation
    Transient Deviation

2. Muscle Examination
   (Tenderness Yes = √)   R   L

    Lateral Pterygoid
    Origin of Masseter
    Insertion of Masseter
    Origin of Temporalis

3. Occlusion
    Angles class
    Is centric occlusion in centric relation?
    If not, premature contact in centric relation?
    Direction of slide:

                               R   L

    Non-working side interference
    Working side interference
    Canine guidance
    Group function
    Cross-over interferences
    Freedom on centric: Yes   No
    Evidence of excessive wear
    Tongue scalloping
    Cheek ridging
    Evidence of enamel/restoration fracture

Flowchart 1 Examination of the articulatory system. **S**1

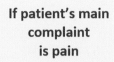

If patient's main
complaint
is pain

First sort out the
source of
the pain

associated mandibular muscle

pain with function

from the joint itself

Pain associated with the masticatory muscles is frequently associated with parafunction

If there are palpable areas of tenderness in the muscles, then physiotherapy has great benefit.

Electrophysiotherapy is thought to have its action by increasing capillary permeability and enhancing the uptake of inflammatory exudate from the tissues surrounding the muscle fibres.

Some modalities of physiotherapy also enhance blood flow.

It is advisable to suggest the patient keeps strictly to a soft diet, such as pasta, mince, fish, eggs, etc. Chewing meat and tearing actions such as biting into crusty French bread and bagels increase the joint load and should be avoided.

Patients should be counselled that biting into something hard with the mouth wide open, such as into an apple, greatly increases the load across the joint and should also be avoided.

Patients should cut up apples and raw vegetables.

Can be associated with an internal disc derangement, degenerative joint disease or an acute inflammatory pain, as is seen with a traumatic arthritis.

Pain may respond to a (NSAID) such as Ibuprofen. If you prescribe this, advise the patient that he/she must take the drug regularly after food for 2—3 days before the anti-inflammatory effect is maximized.

When patients experience intractable pain from advanced degenerative joint disease, intra-articular injection of steroid and local anaesthetic alongside arthrocentesis can be given.

Flowchart 2 The clinical significance of pain. 2

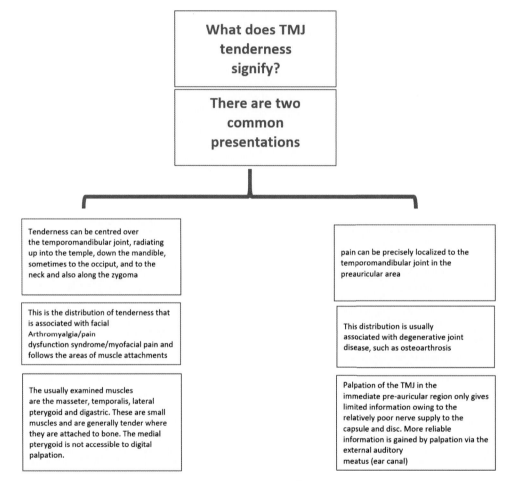

What does TMJ tenderness signify?

There are two common presentations

Tenderness can be centred over the temporomandibular joint, radiating up into the temple, down the mandible, sometimes to the occiput, and to the neck and also along the zygoma

This is the distribution of tenderness that is associated with facial Arthromyalgia/pain dysfunction syndrome/myofacial pain and follows the areas of muscle attachments

The usually examined muscles are the masseter, temporalis, lateral pterygoid and digastric. These are small muscles and are generally tender where they are attached to bone. The medial pterygoid is not accessible to digital palpation.

pain can be precisely localized to the temporomandibular joint in the preauricular area

This distribution is usually associated with degenerative joint disease, such as osteoarthrosis

Palpation of the TMJ in the immediate pre-auricular region only gives limited information owing to the relatively poor nerve supply to the capsule and disc. More reliable information is gained by palpation via the external auditory meatus (ear canal)

Flowchart 3 The clinical significance of TMJ tenderness. 3

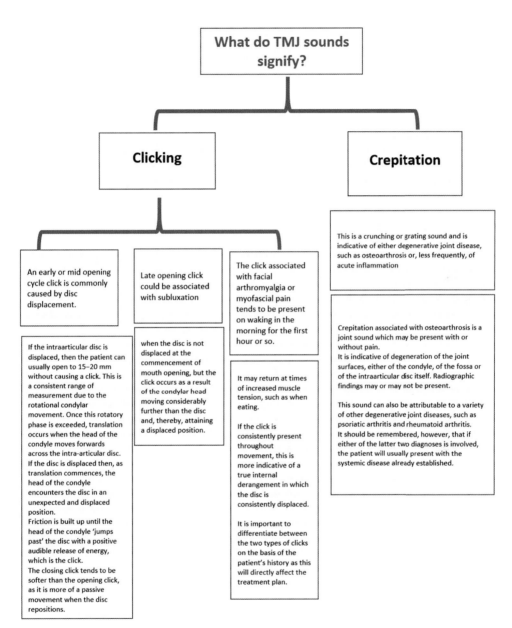

What do TMJ sounds signify?

Clicking

Crepitation

An early or mid opening cycle click is commonly caused by disc displacement.

Late opening click could be associated with subluxation

The click associated with facial arthromyalgia or myofascial pain tends to be present on waking in the morning for the first hour or so.

This is a crunching or grating sound and is indicative of either degenerative joint disease, such as osteoarthrosis or, less frequently, of acute inflammation

If the intraarticular disc is displaced, then the patient can usually open to 15–20 mm without causing a click. This is a consistent range of measurement due to the rotational condylar movement. Once this rotatory phase is exceeded, translation occurs when the head of the condyle moves forwards across the intra-articular disc. If the disc is displaced then, as translation commences, the head of the condyle encounters the disc in an unexpected and displaced position.
Friction is built up until the head of the condyle 'jumps past' the disc with a positive audible release of energy, which is the click.
The closing click tends to be softer than the opening click, as it is more of a passive movement when the disc repositions.

when the disc is not displaced at the commencement of mouth opening, but the click occurs as a result of the condylar head moving considerably further than the disc and, thereby, attaining a displaced position.

It may return at times of increased muscle tension, such as when eating.

If the click is consistently present throughout movement, this is more indicative of a true internal derangement in which the disc is consistently displaced.

It is important to differentiate between the two types of clicks on the basis of the patient's history as this will directly affect the treatment plan.

Crepitation associated with osteoarthrosis is a joint sound which may be present with or without pain.
It is indicative of degeneration of the joint surfaces, either of the condyle, of the fossa or of the intraarticular disc itself. Radiographic findings may or may not be present.

This sound can also be attributable to a variety of other degenerative joint diseases, such as psoriatic arthritis and rheumatoid arthritis. It should be remembered, however, that if either of the latter two diagnoses is involved, the patient will usually present with the systemic disease already established.

Flowchart 4 The clinical significance of TMJ sound. 4

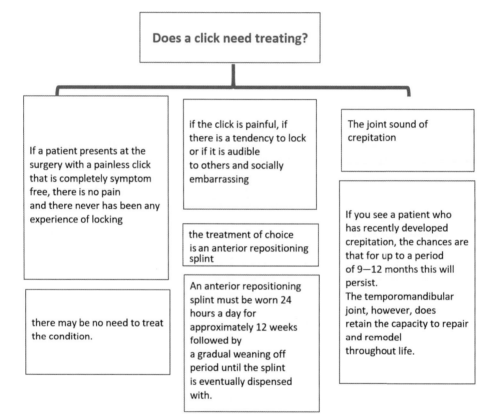

Does a click need treating?

If a patient presents at the surgery with a painless click that is completely symptom free, there is no pain and there never has been any experience of locking

there may be no need to treat the condition.

if the click is painful, if there is a tendency to lock or if it is audible to others and socially embarrassing

the treatment of choice is an anterior repositioning splint

An anterior repositioning splint must be worn 24 hours a day for approximately 12 weeks followed by a gradual weaning off period until the splint is eventually dispensed with.

The joint sound of crepitation

If you see a patient who has recently developed crepitation, the chances are that for up to a period of 9—12 months this will persist.
The temporomandibular joint, however, does retain the capacity to repair and remodel throughout life.

Flowchart 5 Treatment of TMJ sounds. 5

How do I react to a
complaint
of a decreased range of
movement?

Think about the
possible
cause

Muscle Pain

**Internal Derangement of Disc
Displacement,
Without Reduction**

This could be secondary to parafunction,
secondary to trauma or, as happens
frequently, may arise spontaneously with the
patient having done nothing that he/she was
aware of to cause the onset of the symptoms

An intensive course of outpatient physiotherapy, either megapulse
or ultrasound, directed at 'relaxing' the superior pterygoid muscle,
to be helpful
If this is of recent onset, there is a high chance of success of allowing
the disc to reposition.
This must be an intensive course (3x per week for 3 weeks).

NSAIDs, such as Ibuprofen, do have a place. A
more effective way of addressing this,
however, is with an immediate and intensive
course of outpatient electro-physiotherapy in
combination with a soft diet and anti-
inflammatory gel, preferably containing both
Ibuprofen and Levomenthol.

If the disc displacement is recent and associated with acute muscle
spasm of the superior pterygoid, then prescription of Temazepam
oral suspension should also be considered. This must be done in
conjunction with the patient's medical practitioner and should be
given as a 10 mg dose at night for a period of about 10–12 days.
The patient should be counselled to take this half an hour before
going to sleep at night. The dose must not be increased beyond
10 mg and ideally should be gradually reduced. This drug is not
licensed as a muscle relaxant but as an anxiolytic.

It does, however, have a recognized pharmacological muscle
relaxant effect. It is not licensed for use in children under 12
years of age.

When the pain is acute, hot and cold
compresses can be used, such as frozen peas
for a minute wrapped up in a towel followed
by a hot water bottle for 2–3 minutes,
repeating this cycle two or three
times.

If locking is of very recent onset, it is sometimes possible to manipulate the
mandible to free the disc. This is done by asking the patient to bite with a
wooden tongue spatula between the molar teeth on the affected side for
approximately one minute. This causes the muscles on the contra-lateral
side to pull the condyle up while the condyle on the affected side is 'fixed'.
The patient is then asked to open the mouth gently and the operator places
his/ her thumbs on the molar teeth and exerts gentle downwards and
posterior pressure on the affected side, while rotating the other side
upwards and slightly forwards.
This does work on occasion in freeing the disc but the patient should be told
that the disc is unstable. This must be followed by a period of a strict soft
diet and reduction of mouth opening as far as possible.

If a patient presents with a specific area of
acute muscle spasm, which is readily
identifiable by digital palpation, a
vapo-coolant spray, such as ethyl chloride
can be used for temporary relief.

This should be administered in the
surgery environment.

Flowchart 6 The clinical significance of decreased range of movement. 6

Splint Therapy

Soft bite guard soft poly-vinyl vacuum formed appliance	Stabilisation Splint (SS)	Anterior Repositioning Splint (ARPS)
Has limited value. Some patients who use these get better but they possibly represent the group of patients who would get better anyway as their symptoms are self-limiting. In a percentage of patients these appliances can make symptoms worse as the patient is so aware of having something compressible between the teeth that this increases parafunction.	A high clinical success rate of SS therapy in reducing signs and symptoms of myofascial pain has been reported. The long-term success rate of SS has been demonstrated in several studies and there is no need in the overwhelming majority of patients for 'second phase' permanent alteration of the patient's occlusion either by means of orthodontic treatment or by advanced restorative treatment.	This splint was found to be highly successful in reducing or eliminating TMJ clicking when it could be demonstrated at the chairside that the click was eliminated by asking the patient to open and close from a protruded position. On occasion when the patient does this it is painful and/or the click becomes worse and in these circumstances ARPS treatment is not advised. ARPS is an appropriate treatment for patients suffering from disc displacement with reduction provided that it is used for 24 hours a day throughout the treatment period Splint therapy should be stopped immediately if any of the splint fractures leaving some teeth uncovered and thereby changing it into a partial coverage appliance.

Flowchart 7 Splint therapy in the management of TMDs. 7

'The triple-P approch'

Plates

occlusal appliances, most commonly of the hard acrylic resin occlusal stabilization splint type. These appliances probably function more like protectors of the remaining teeth rather than that they actually diminish the bruxism behaviour

Pep talk

stands for **counselling, a behavioural approach** that includes addressing the patient's awareness of the movement disorder, relaxation and lifestyle and sleep hygiene instructions. Albeit of unproven efficacy, these approaches can be applied safely in bruxism patients

Pills

represents **pharmacological interventions** with centrally acting drugs such as benzodiazepines. As long as definitive evidence is missing, the use of medicines in the treatment of bruxism should be confined to short periods and to severe cases in which occlusal appliances and counselling were ineffective. Such approach should be performed in close collaboration with medical specialists.

Flowchart 8 The suggested Triple-P approach in the management of bruxism. (Lobbezoo, F., Van Der Zaag, J., Van Selms, M.K.A., Hamburger, H.L. and Naeije, M. (2008), Principles for the management of bruxism*. Journal of Oral Rehabilitation, 35: 509–523. © 2008, John Wiley & Sons.) Ⓢ8

---

1. **Distribution**
   Localised (1 or 2 sextants)
   Generalised (3-6 sextants)

2. **Severity**
   Mild (wear within the enamel; occlusal/incisal and/or non-occlusal /non-incisal)
   Moderate (wear within dentin exposure; occlusal/incisal and /or non-occlusal/non-incisal)
   Severe (wear within dentin exposure and loss of clinical crown height < 2/3 occlusal/incisal; regardless of the non-occlusal/non-incisal wear)
   Extreme (wear with dentin exposure and loss of clinical crown height ≥ 2/3 occlusal/incisal; regardless of the non-occlusal/incisal; regardless of the non-occlusal/non-incisal wear)

3. **Origin**
   Mechanical/intrinsic (attrition)
   Mechanical/extrinsic (abrasion)
   Chemical/intrinsic (erosion)
   Chemical/extrinsic (erosion)

Flowchart 9 A proposal for the classification of toothwear (Wetselaar and Lobbezoo 2018.) *(Examples of diagnoses are localised severe tooth wear (sextant 2), mainly chemical/intrinsic; generalised moderate tooth wear (sextants 1, 3, 4 and 6), partial mechanical/intrinsic, and partial chemical/ intrinsic; and generalised extreme tooth wear (all sextants), mainly chemical/extrinsic and partial mechanical/extrinsic)*

9

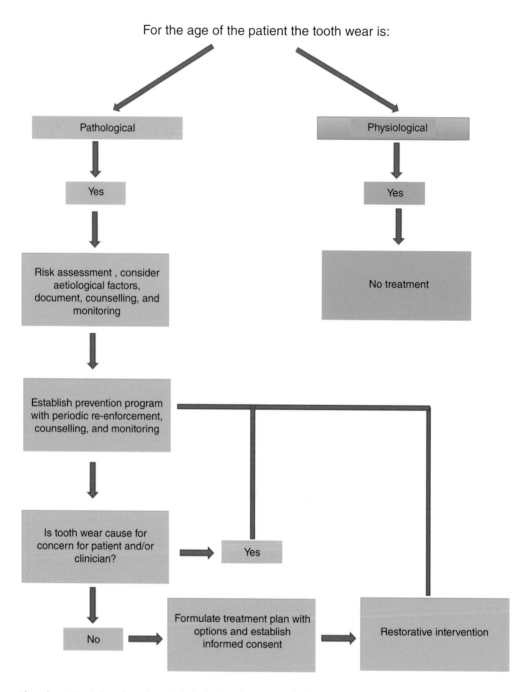

For the age of the patient the tooth wear is:

Pathological

Physiological

Yes

Yes

Risk assessment , consider aetiological factors, document, counselling, and monitoring

No treatment

Establish prevention program with periodic re-enforcement, counselling, and monitoring

Is tooth wear cause for concern for patient and/or clinician?

Yes

No

Formulate treatment plan with options and establish informed consent

Restorative intervention

Flowchart 10 A flowchart that might help the clinician make the appropriate decision and give treatment advice, from counselling and monitoring towards restorative treatment. (Loomans B, Opdam N, Attin T, et al. 2017, Severe Tooth Wear: European Consensus Statement on Management Guidelines. J Adhes Dent; 19(2): 111–119. © 2017, Quintessenz.) 10

Site – Where is the pain? Or the maximal site of the pain.

Onset – When did the pain start, and was it sudden or gradual? Include also whether it is progressive or regressive.

Character –What is the pain like? An ache? Stabbing?

Radiation – Does the pain radiate anywhere?

Associations – Any other signs or symptom associated with the pain?

Time course – Does the pain follow any pattern?

Exacerbating/relieving factors – Does anything change the pain?

Severity – How bad is the pain?

Flowchart 11 SOCRATES is a good mnemonic for remembering the different questions to ask when presented pain.

How should orthodontic treatment be managed if the patient presents signs and symptoms of TMD before or during treatment?

- Before starting orthodontic treatment, it is advisable to perform always a screening examination for the presence of TMD.
- For medico-legal reasons, any findings, including TMJ sounds, deviation during mandibular movements or pain, should be recorded and updated at 6-month intervals.
- Informed consent should be signed by the patient.
- If the patient presents signs or symptoms of TMD before starting orthodontic treatment, the first step is to make the diagnosis.
- When the patient's chief complaint is pain, it is important to make a differential diagnosis to determine whether the pain is because of TMD, i.e. musculoskeletal condition, or to another disease.
- Resolve the pain by following a conservative treatment protocol including pharmacotherapy, counselling, behavioural therapy, home exercises, physical therapy and / or occlusal appliances.
- Orthodontic treatment should not be initiated as long as a patient suffers from facial pain.
- Once the pain has been resolved and the condition is stable over a reasonable amount of time, initiation of orthodontic therapy may be considered.
- TMD signs and symptoms are fluctuating and unpredictable and can emerge during orthodontic treatment. The orthodontist should inform the patient about that
- Orthodontic treatment has to be performed according to the rules that allow an 'ideal and stable' result to be achieved.

Flowchart 12 How should orthodontic treatment be managed if the patient presents signs and symptoms of TMD before or during treatment? (Michelotti A, Iodice G. 2010, The role of orthodontics in temporomandibular disorders. J Oral Rehabil; 37(6): 411–429. © 2010, John Wiley & Sons.) 12

Checklist of essential criteria required by TMD specialist

Presenting Complaint

1. Patient's prime complaint or dentist's concern   ☑

History of presenting complaint

2. Length of time complaint has been present   ☑

3. Frequency of presenting complaint   ☑

4. Change in signs or symptoms noted   ☑

5. Any event associated with onset of problem   ☑

6. Qualification of prime signs and symptoms   ☑

7. Exacerbating factors   ☑

8. Relieving factors   ☑

9. Previous treatment   ☑

10. Other factors   ☑

11. Relevant medical history

12. Relevant social history   ☑

13. Examination details   ☑

14. Provisional diagnosis suggested   ☑

15. Offer to treat   ☑

16. GDP states what she/she requests   ☑

VERY HELPFUL   (13–16)
SOME HELP   (5–12)
VERY LITTLE HELP (0–4)

Flowchart 13 Checklist of essential criteria required by TMD specialist. (O'Donovan et al 2003.) **Ⓢ**13

Appendix II

Glossary of Terms

This glossary contains not only terms used in this text but also other terms that the reader might find useful. Think of this section not so much as a glossary but more as a dictionary.

Abfraction — the pathological loss of hard tooth substance caused by biomechanical loading forces.

Acupuncture — the use of a needle, either electrically stimulated or not, inserted into an acupuncture tract or an irritable focus in a soft-tissue structure, most commonly muscle.

Adhesion — (1) the stable joining of parts to each other, which may occur abnormally; (2) a fibrous band or structure by which parts abnormally adhere.

Adhesive capsulitis — within the temporomandibular joint, any situation in which the disc is in its normal position, the joint space volume is decreased, and motion is restricted

Angle's classification of occlusion — eponym for a classification system of occlusion based on the interdigitation of the first molar teeth, originally described by Angle as four major groups depending on the antero-posterior jaw relationship.

Ankylosis — joint immobility, either bony or fibrous, due to injury, disease or surgery.

Anterior band of the intra-articular disc — a component of the intra-articular disc interposed between the head of the condyle and the articular eminence at maximum opening.

Anterior bite plane — an individually fabricated anterior guide table that allows mandibular movement without the influence of tooth contact and facilitates the recording of maxillo-mandibular relationships.

Anterior deprogrammer — see anterior bite plane.

Anterior disc displacement — see disc displacement.

Temporomandibular Disorders: A Problem-Based Approach, Second Edition. M. Ziad Al-Ani and Robin J.M. Gray.
© 2021 M. Ziad Al-Ani and Robin J.M. Gray. Published 2021 by John Wiley & Sons Ltd.
Companion Website: www.wiley.com/go/al-ani/temporomandibular-disorders-2e

Anterior guidance — guidance of the mandible during eccentric movements as provided by occlusal contacts. See also ideal anterior guidance; posterior guidance.

Anterior repositioning splint (ARPS) — an appliance to guide the mandible to a rest position from which the patient can open 'click free' because the disc displacement has reduced.

Arthralgia — pain in a joint or joints.

Arthrocentesis — a technique used to treat some cases of osteoarthritic TMJ which involves introduction of a cannula into the joint space to perform joint irrigation, with two needles within the joint space to allow continual flow of fluid in and out. Medications, such as local anaesthetics, steroids, and synthetic synovial fluids, may be added during arthrocentesis. The lavage is thought to eliminate much of the secondary inflammatory mediators that produce pain.

Arthrodial joint — a joint that allows gliding motion of the surfaces.

Arthrodial movement — gliding joint movement.

Arthrography — radiological investigation involving introduction of opaque contrast medium into one (or both) temporomandibular joint space, performed to determine disc position or perforation.

Arthropathy — a disease of a joint.

Arthroplasty — the surgical formation or reformation of a joint.

Arthroscopy of TMJ — involves placing an arthroscope into the superior joint space, rendering the intracapsular structures visible on a monitor. Bone spurs can be removed with shavers and the joint space can be increased by inflation of balloon stents. This procedure has been shown to be successful in reducing symptoms and improving the range of jaw movement in patients with TMJ osteoarthrosis. Therapeutic agents can also be placed using this technique.

Arthrosis — a degenerative disease of a joint.

Articular — of or relating to a joint.

Articular cartilage — a thin layer of hyaline cartilage located on the joint surfaces of some bones; not found on the articular surfaces of the temporomandibular joints, that are covered with an avascular fibrous tissue.

Articular disc — see intra-articular disc.

Articular eminence — the anterior slope of the glenoid fossa, down which the condyle moves during mouth opening.

Articulate — (1) to join together as a joint; (2) the relating of contacting surfaces of the teeth or their artificial replicas in the maxillae to those in the mandible

Articulating paper — ink-coated paper strips used to locate and mark occlusal contacts.

Articulating surfaces — the fibrous tissue covered surfaces of both the mandibular condyle and glenoid fossa.

Articulation — the place of union or junction between two or more bones of the skeleton. In dentistry, the static and dynamic contact relationship between the occlusal surfaces of the teeth during function.

Articulator — a mechanical instrument that represents the temporo-mandibular joints and jaws, to which maxillary and mandibular casts may be attached to simulate some or all mandibular movements.

Articulatory system — comprises the temporomandibular joints, masticatory muscles, occlusion.

Attrition — the act of wearing or grinding down by friction, or mechanical wear resulting from mastication or parafunction, limited to contacting surfaces of the teeth.

Atypical facial pain — a dull aching or throbbing pain, the distribution of which does not follow the established pathways of innervation of the major sensory nerves. A clinical examination seldom reveals any abnormalities.

Auscultation — the process of determining the condition of various parts of the body by listening to the sounds that they emit.

Autologous blood injection — or autohemotherapy, comprises certain types of hemotherapy using a person's own blood.

Autopolymerising resin — a resin, the polymerization of which is initiated by a chemical activator.

Average value articulator — an articulator that is fabricated to permit motion based on mean mandibular movements – also called class III articulator

Axial loading — the force directed down the long axis of a body usually used to describe the force of occlusal contact on a natural tooth, dental implant or other object; axial loading is best described as the force down the long axis of the tooth or whatever body is being described.

Balanced articulation — the bilateral, simultaneous, anterior and posterior occlusal contact of teeth in centric and eccentric positions.

Balancing side — see non-working side.

Benzodiazepine — a group of hypnotic and anxiolytic drugs that, in small doses, have a pharmacological muscle relaxant effect.

Bilaminar zone — a mass of loose, highly vascular, and highly innervated connective tissue attached to the posterior edge of the articular disc, and extending to and filling the loose folds of the posterior capsule of the temporomandibular joint; also called retrodiscal tissue.

Bilateral balanced articulation — also termed balanced articulation, the bilateral, simultaneous anterior and posterior occlusal contact of teeth in centric and eccentric positions.

Bimanual manipulation technique — a method for placement of the mandible using both thumbs on the chin and the fingers on the inferior border of the mandible to guide the jaw into centric relation.

Bimanual palpation — a technique of muscle examination, using both hands.

Biofeedback — a means of providing a patient with audible or visual information, enabling him or her to gain a degree of voluntary control over the function under examination.

Bite — see occlusion.

Bite of convenience — see centric occlusion.

Border movement — mandibular movement at the limits dictated by anatomical structures, as viewed in a given plane.

Botulinum toxins — (Botox) is a neurotoxic protein produced by the bacterium *Clostridium botulinum* and related species. It prevents the release of the neurotransmitter acetylcholine from axon endings at the neuromuscular junction and thus causes flaccid paralysis.

Bruxism — a habitual tooth grinding activity. See also parafunction.

Canine guidance — an example of an ideal anterior guidance, in which the upper canine exclusively provides the guidance during mandibular lateral excursion.

Canine protected occlusion — see canine guidance.

Capsule — fibrous tissue, lined by synovial membrane, that encloses the joint and limits joint movement.

Cartilage — a derivative of connective tissue arising from the mesenchyme. Typical hyaline cartilage is a flexible, rather elastic, material with a semi-transparent glass-like appearance. Its ground substance is a complex protein through which there is distributed a large network of connective tissue fibres.

Centric occlusion (CO) — the static tooth relationship into which patients habitually close their teeth.

Centric relation (CR) — a reproducible jaw position, independent of tooth contact, which conceptually is the position of the mandible relative to the skull when the muscles are at their most relaxed and in a least strained position. Anatomically, the disc must be in place and the head of the condyle in its most superior position and in the terminal hinge axis.

Centric relation appliance — see stabilisation splint.

Centric relation occlusion — this is the occlusion when the teeth meet evenly without any premature contacts in the centric relation jaw position. See also centric occlusion; centric relation.

Centric relation record — a registration of the relationship of the maxilla to the mandible when the mandible is in centric relation.

Centric slide — the movement of the mandible while in centric relation, from the initial occlusal contact into maximum intercuspation.

Cheek ridging — ridging of the buccal mucosa, usually along the occlusal plane; taken as a sign of active bruxism.

Chronic pain — pain marked by long duration or frequent recurrence.

Clenching — a habitual contraction of masticatory elevator muscles when the teeth are together and independent of normal function, often resulting in muscle symptoms. See also parafunction.

Click — a brief, sharp audible release of energy within the joint thought to be caused by the sudden distraction of opposing wet surfaces.

Clicking — a series of clicks, such as the snapping, cracking or noise evident on excursions of the mandible; a distinct snapping sound or sensation, usually detectable on palpation or by stethoscope, which emanates from the temporomandibular joint(s) during jaw movement. It may or may not be associated with internal derangements of the temporomandibular joint.

Closed lock — intercuspation TMJ locking.

Computed tomography — a method of imaging using X-rays that allows the production of cross-sectional images of hard and soft tissues.

Condylar aplasia — developmental defect resulting in an absence of the mandibular condyle. Rare condition that may produce facial asymmetry.

Condylar axis — a hypothetical line through the mandibular condyles around which the mandible may rotate.

Condylar dislocation — a non-self-reducing displacement of the mandibular condyle, usually forward of the articular eminence.

Condylar guidance — mandibular guidance generated by the condyle and articular disc traversing the contour of the glenoid fossae.

Condylar guide assembly — the components of an articulator that guide movement of the condylar analogues.

Condylar guide inclination — the angle formed by the inclination of a condylar guide control surface of an articulator and a specified reference plane.

Condylar hinge position — the position of the condyles of the mandible in the glenoid fossae, at which hinge axis movement is possible.

Condylar hyperplasia — although rare, the most common of the developmental defects affecting the mandibular condyle. It is usually unilateral and associated with facial asymmetry and altered occlusion.

Condylar hypoplasia — incomplete or under-development of the head of the mandibular condyle. Rare condition that may produce facial asymmetry.

Condylar inclination — the direction of the lateral condyle path.

Condylar path element — the member of a dental articulator that controls the direction of condylar movement.

Condylar subluxation — a self-reducing incomplete or partial dislocation of the condyle.

Condyle — in the mandible, the projection of bone that articulates with the glenoid fossa.

Condylectomy — surgical removal of the condyle.

Condylotomy — surgical cut through the neck of the condyloid process; also refers to surgical removal of a portion of the articulating surface of the mandibular condyle (called a condylar shave).

Connective tissue — a tissue of mesodermal origin, rich in interlacing processes, that supports or binds together other tissues.

Coronoid maxillary space — the region between the medial aspect of the coronoid process of the mandible and the buccal aspect of the tuberosity of the maxilla, bounded anteriorly by the zygomatic arch.

Coronoid process — the thin, triangular, rounded eminence originating from the anterosuperior surface of the ramus of the mandible.

Craniocervical mandibular syndrome — see pain dysfunction syndrome.

Craniomandibular articulation — both temporomandibular joints functioning together as a bilateral sliding hinge joint connecting the mandible to the cranium.

Craniomandibular dysfunction — see pain dysfunction syndrome.

Crepitus — the 'grating' joint sound throughout jaw movement, characteristic of degenerative joint disease.

Crossover interference — a posterior interference when the mandible has reached or exceeded the canine crossover position. See also posterior interference; crossover position.

Crossover position — the position during lateral mandibular excursion; when in a class I or II occlusion, the mandibular canine is labial to the maxillary canine.

Dahl concept — this describes a method of creating inter-occlusal space in a localised part of the mouth not only to enable placement of restorations on worn teeth but also has use in a variety of other clinical situations.

Decreased occlusal vertical dimension — a reduction in the distance measured between two anatomic points when the teeth are in occlusal contact.

Deflective occlusal contact — a contact that displaces a tooth or diverts the mandible from its intended movement. See also occlusal disharmony, occlusal prematurity.

Degenerative joint disease — see osteoarthrosis.

Dental panoramic tomogram (DPT) — a scanning radiograph showing the dental tissues and associated bones. A modified projection can image the head of condyle.

Deviation of mandibular movement — during opening or closing of the mandible, a discursive movement that may be lasting or transient.

Diagnostic cast — a life-size reproduction of a part of the oral cavity for the purpose of study and treatment planning.

Diagnostic occlusal adjustment — an evaluation of the process and implications of subtractive tooth adjustment on articulator-mounted casts, for the determination of the benefits and consequences of an occlusal adjustment.

Diarthrodial joint — a joint with two separate movements and two joint compartments. The temporomandibular joints are diarthrodial synovial paired joints.

Direction of slide — direction of mandibular movement when moving from the first contact in centric relation to maximum intercuspation in centric occlusion. See also centric relation; centric occlusion; premature contact.

Disc — see intra-articular disc.

Disc displacement with reduction — a derangement in which the disc displacement (usually anteromedially) is not maintained, the disc repositioning to a normal functional position during opening, causing the clinical sign of clicking.

Disc displacement without reduction — a derangement in which the disc displacement (usually anteromedially) is maintained during opening, causing the clinical sign of locking.

Disc perforation — a defect in the intra-articular disc, usually in the posterior part, allowing communication between upper and lower joint spaces. It generally results from degenerative thinning in the central portion, usually with longstanding increased compressive forces or as a result of trauma. There is no disruption at the peripheral attachments to the capsule, ligaments or bone.

Disc thinning — degenerative decrease in disc thickness, usually as the result of longstanding increased compressive forces.

Disc–condyle complex — the condyle and its disc articulation.

Discectomy — excision of the intra-articular disc.

Dislocation — an unusual condition in which the head of the condyle sublux-ates beyond the articular eminence; the resultant muscle pull (upwards and backwards) prevents mouth closure.

Dynamic occlusion — the contacts between the teeth when the mandible is moving relative to the maxilla.

Dysfunction — a collective term of signs and symptoms of an abnormal or altered function.

Earbow — an instrument similar to a facebow that indexes the external auditory meatus and registers the relation of the maxillary dental arch to the external auditory meatus and a horizontal reference plane. This instrument is used to transfer the maxillary cast to the articulator. The earbow provides an average anatomical dimension between the external auditory meatus and the horizontal axis of the mandible. See also facebow.

Eccentric mandibular movement — an excursive movement of the mandible relative to the maxilla from centric occlusion.

Elastic attachment of the intra-articular disc — the upper attachment of the posterior bilaminar zone of the intra-articular disc to the fossa, at the level of the squamotympanic fissure.

Equilibration — a demanding clinical procedure in which permanent and irreversible changes are made to the patient's natural dentition, with the objective of providing a more ideal occlusion.

Excursive movements — see lateral excursion; protrusion.

Facebow — a device used in mounting the maxillary cast in a semi-adjustable articulator by recording the relationship between the maxillary teeth and the estimated condylar position.

Facebow fork — that component of the facebow used to attach the occlusal rim to the facebow.

Facebow record — the registration obtained by means of a facebow.

Facebow transfer — the process of transferring the facebow record of the spatial relationship of the maxillary arch to some anatomical reference point(s) and transferring this relationship to an articulator.

Facet (wear facet) — an area on a tooth or restoration worn down by attrition.

Facial arthromyalgia — see myofascial pain.

Fibrous adhesion — a fibrous band or structure by which parts abnormally adhere.

Fibrous ankylosis — reduced mobility of a joint due to proliferation of fibrous tissue.

Fibrous attachment — the lower attachments of the posterior bilaminar zone of the intra-articular disc of the neck of the condyle.

Fossa — an anatomical pit, groove, or depression.

Fox appliance — see stabilisation splint.

Freedom in centric (long centric) — freedom in centric occlusion occurs when the mandible can move anteriorly for a small distance in the same horizontal and sagittal plane while maintaining tooth contact.

Fully adjustable articulator — an articulator that allows replication of three-dimensional movement of recorded mandibular motion – also called a class IV articulator.

Functional mandibular movements — all normal, proper, or characteristic movements of the mandible made during speech, mastication, yawning, swallowing, and other associated movements.

Functional occlusal harmony — the occlusal relationship of opposing teeth in all functional ranges and movements that will provide the greatest masticatory efficiency without causing undue strain or trauma on the supporting tissues.

Functional occlusal splint — a device that directs the movements of the mandible by controlling the plane and range of motion.

Functional occlusion — the contacts of the maxillary and mandibular teeth during mastication and deglutition.

Glenoid fossa — the concavity in the temporal bone by the zygomatic arch that receives the mandibular condyle.

Gliding movement — see translation.

Group function — an example of an ideal anterior guidance in which usually the maxillary canine, premolar and even the buccal cusps of the first molars provide the guidance during lateral excursions of the mandible. The earliest and hardest contacts are provided towards the front of the group.

Guidance — providing regulation or direction to movement; a guide – the influence on mandibular movements by the contacting surfaces of the maxillary and mandibular anterior teeth; mechanical forms on the lower anterior portion of an articulator that guide movements of its upper member. *See* anterior guidance; condylar guidance.

Habitual bite — see centric occlusion.

Hinge axis — an imaginary line around which the mandible may rotate within the sagittal plane.

Hyperactivity — excessive motor activity.

Hyperplasia — the abnormal multiplication or increase in the number of normal cells in normal arrangement in a tissue.

Hypertonicity — increased resting muscle activity resulting in an excessive contractile state.

Iatrogenic — resulting from the activity of the clinician; applied to disorders induced in the patient by the clinician.

Ideal anterior guidance — canine guidance or group function with posterior disclusion. See also ideal occlusion; anterior guidance; posterior guidance.

Ideal occlusion — a centric occlusion that occurs in centric relation from which excentric movements of the mandible can occur with anterior guidance at the front of the mouth and with posterior disclusion. See also canine guidance; centric occlusion; centric relation; group function; ideal anterior guidance; posterior interference.

Imaging techniques — techniques for assessing bony and, on occasions soft-tissue structures which include – plain radiography and tomography; arthrography; computed tomography; magnetic resonance imaging; and scintigraphy.

Incisal guidance — the influence of the contacting surfaces of the mandibular and maxillary anterior teeth on mandibular movements; the influences of the contacting surfaces of the guide pin and guide table on articulator movements.

Incisal guide angle — anatomically, the angle formed by the intersection of the plane of occlusion and a line within the sagittal plane determined by the incisal edges of the maxillary and mandibular central incisors, when the teeth are in maximum intercuspation. On an articulator, that angle formed, in the sagittal plane, between the plane of reference and the slope of the anterior guide table, as viewed in the sagittal plane.

Incisal opening — a measurement of mouth opening taken from incisor tip to incisor tip. Usually recorded at both a 'pain-free' and 'maximal' opening levels.

Inferior pterygoid — inferior head of lateral pterygoid muscle inserted into the anterior aspect of the neck of the condyles. Active in mouth opening. See also lateral pterygoid.

Infraocclusion — occlusion in which the occluding surfaces of teeth are below the normal plane of occlusion.

Initial occlusal contact — during closure of the mandible, the first or initial contact of opposing teeth between the arches.

Intercondylar distance — the distance between the rotational centres of two condyles or their analogues.

Intercuspal contact — the contact between the cusps of opposing teeth.

Intercuspal contact area — the range of tooth contacts in maximum intercuspation.

Intercuspation position (ICP) — a synonym for centric occlusion.

Interference — in dentistry, any tooth contacts that interfere with or hinder harmonious mandibular movement.

Intermediate zone of the intra-articular disc — a component of the intra-articular disc interposed between the head of the condyle and the articular eminence during the translatory phase of opening.

Internal derangement — structural defect or abnormal position of tissues within the capsule of the joint (usually involving disc displacement) which interferes with smooth joint movement.

Interocclusal — between the occlusal surfaces of opposing teeth.

Interocclusal clearance — the arrangement in which the opposing occlusal surfaces may pass each other without any contact; the amount of reduction achieved during tooth preparation to provide for an adequate thickness of restorative material.

Interocclusal distance — the distance between the occluding surfaces of the maxillary and mandibular teeth when the mandible is in a specified position.

Interocclusal gap — see interocclusal distance.

Interocclusal record — a registration of the positional relationship of the opposing teeth or arches; a record of the positional relationship of the teeth or jaws to each other.

Interocclusal rest space — the difference between the vertical dimension at rest and the vertical dimension while in occlusion.

Intra-articular disc — sheet of dense fibrous tissue, interposed between the head of condyle and the glenoid fossa, which is divided into four zones.

Intracapsular adhesion — adhesions occurring within the joint capsule, resulting in reduced mobility.

Intracapsular ankylosis — diminished joint motion due to disease, injury or surgical procedure within a joint capsule.

Intracapsular disorder — a problem associated with the masticatory system in which the aetiological factors are located within the temporomandibular joint capsule.

Intracapsular fracture — a fracture of the condyle of the mandible occurring within the confines of the capsule of the temporomandibular joint – also called intra-articular fracture.

Intracondylar — within the condyle.

Jig — a device used to maintain mechanically the correct positional relationship between a piece of work and a tool, or between components during assembly or alteration.

Kinematic axis — the transverse horizontal axis connecting the rotational centres of the right and left condyles.

Kinematic facebow — a facebow with adjustable calliper ends used to locate the transverse horizontal axis of the mandible.

Kinematics — the phase of mechanics that deals with the possible motions of a material body.

Laser — acronym for light amplification by simulated emission of radiation; a device that transforms light of various frequencies into an intense, small and almost non-divergent beam of monochromatic radiation, within the visible range.

Laser therapy — a method of electrophysiotherapy, which produces a non-thermal response in the tissues but increases blood flow.

Lasting mandibular deviation — a mandibular pathway where the mandible moves vertically during the first phase of movement and then has an abrupt lateral deviation, this could imply that there is disc displacement without reduction.

Late closing click — the sound emanating from the temporomandibular joint that occurs just before termination of closure in patients with an anteriorly displaced disc.

Late opening click — the sound emanating from the temporomandibular joint that occurs just before termination of opening in patients with an anteriorly displaced disc.

Lateral condylar inclination — the angle formed by the path of the moving condyle within the horizontal plane compared with the median plane (antero-posterior movement) and within the frontal plane when compared with the horizontal plane (superoinferior movement).

Lateral condylar path — the path of movement of the condyle–disc assembly in the joint cavity when a lateral mandibular movement is made.

Lateral excursion — movement of the mandible relative to the maxilla, primarily in the right or left lateral direction.

Lateral ligament — a thickening of the fibrous tissue of the lateral part of the joint capsule.

Lateral pterygoid muscle — a muscle originating from the lateral surface of the lateral pterygoid plate and the infratemporal surface of the greater wing of the sphenoid bone, and inserting by two independent heads (superior pterygoid/inferior pterygoid) into the intra-articular disc and neck of the condyle, respectively. See also superior pterygoid; inferior pterygoid.

Laterodetrusion — lateral and downward movement of the condyle on the working side.

Lateroprotrusion — a protrusive movement of the mandibular condyle in which there is a lateral component.

Lateroretrusion — lateral and backward movement of the condyle on the working side.

Laterosurtrusion — lateral and upward movement of the condyle on the working side.

Laterotrusion — condylar movement on the working side in the horizontal plane. This term may be used in combination with terms describing condylar movement in other planes, e.g. laterodetrusion, lateroprotrusion, lateroretrusion, and laterosurtrusion.

Localised occlusal interference splint (LOIS) — an appliance designed to interfere with the occlusion and deter bruxism.

Locking of TMJ — see TMJ locking.

Long centric — see freedom in centric.

Lucia jig — an individually fabricated anterior guide table that allows mandibular motion without the influence of tooth contacts, and facilitates the recording of maxillomandibular relationships.

Luxation — an abnormal anterior displacement of the mandibular condyle out of the glenoid fossa that is self-reducing.

Magnetic resonance imaging (MRI) — a method of imaging using non-ionising radiation, in which the patient is placed in a large magnetic field and exposed to radio waves. Cross-sectional images of hard and soft tissues are produced.

Malocclusion — any deviation from a physiologically acceptable contact between the opposing dental arches; any deviation from a normal occlusion.

Mandibular dislocation — a non-self-reducing displacement of the mandibular condyle out of the glenoid fossa.

Mandibular dysfunction — see myofascial pain.

Mandibular hinge position — the position of the mandible in relation to the maxilla, at which opening and closing movements occur on the hinge axis.

Mandibular stress syndrome — see myofascial pain.

Manipulation under anaesthetic — a non-surgical procedure carried out under a general anaesthetic with the intention of increasing a hitherto limited range of mandibular movement.

Masseter muscle — a muscle originating from the inferior aspect of the anterior two-thirds of the zygomatic arch and inserting into the lateral aspect of the angle of the mandible. In normal function, one of the principal elevator muscles of the mandible.

Masticating cycles — the patterns of mandibular movements formed during the chewing of food.

Mastication — the process of chewing food for swallowing and digestion.

Masticatory apparatus — see masticatory system.

Masticatory cycle — a three-dimensional representation of mandibular movement produced during the chewing of food.

Masticatory efficiency — the effort required in achieving a standard degree of comminution.

Masticatory force — the force applied by the muscles of mastication during chewing.

Masticatory movements — mandibular movements used for chewing food. See also masticatory cycle.

Masticatory muscle disorder — see myofascial pain.

Masticatory muscles — muscles that elevate the mandible to close the mouth (temporalis, superficial and deep masseter, and medial pterygoid).

Masticatory myalgia — see myofascial pain.

Masticatory pain — discomfort about the face and mouth induced by chewing or other use of the jaws, but independent of local disease involving the teeth and mouth.

Masticatory performance — a measure of the comminution of food attainable under standardised testing conditions.

Masticatory system — comprises the teeth, periodontal tissues and articulatory system.

Maxillomandibular registration — see maxillomandibular relationship record.

Maxillomandibular relationship — any spatial relationship of the maxillae to the mandible; any one of the infinite relationships of the mandible to the maxillae.

Maxillomandibular relationship record — a registration of any positional relationship of the mandible relative to the maxillae. These records may be made at any vertical, horizontal or lateral orientation.

Maximal intercuspal contacts — tooth contact in the maximum intercuspal position.

Maximal intercuspal position — the complete intercuspation of the opposing teeth independent of condylar position, sometimes referred to as the best fit of the teeth regardless of the condylar position – also called maximal intercuspation. See centric occlusion.

Meatus — a natural body passage; a general term for any opening or passageway in the body.

Medial pterygoid — a muscle originating from between the pterygoid plates and inserting into medial aspect of the angle of the mandible. In normal function, active in closing and excursive movements of the mandible.

Mediotrusion — a movement of the condyle medially. See also non-working side.

Megapulse — pulsed short-wave diathermy, the rest period allowing for dissipation of heat by the blood flow. See also short-wave diathermy.

Meniscectomy — excision of the intra-articular disc. See also discectomy.

Meniscus — see intra-articular disc.

Michigan splint — see stabilisation splint.

Microtrauma — minor injury, which, if repetitive, may cause damage.

Mid-opening click — the abnormal sound emanating from the temporomandibular joint that occurs during midprotrusive translation of the condyles.

Migraine — an idiopathic recurring headache disorder typically lasting 4–72 hours, may be with or without aura and associated with nausea and photo-and phonophobia.

Muscle contraction — the shortening and development of tension in a muscle in response to stimulation.

Muscle contracture — a condition of high resistance to passive stretching of a muscle, resulting from fibrosis of the tissues supporting the muscle or the joint; sustained increased resistance to passive stretch with reduced muscle length.

Muscle hyperalgesia — increased sensitivity to pain in a muscle evoked by stimulation at the site of pain in the muscle.

Muscle hypertension — increased muscular tension that is not easily released but does not prevent normal lengthening of the muscles involved.

Muscle hypertonicity — increased contractile activity in some motor units driven by reflex arcs from receptors in the muscle and/or α motoneurons of the spinal cord.

Muscle relaxant — a drug or therapy that diminishes muscle tension.

Muscle spasm — a sudden involuntary contraction of a muscle or group of muscles attended by pain and interference with function. It differs from muscle splinting in that the contraction is sustained even when the muscle is at rest, and the pain/dysfunction is present with passive and active movements of the affected part – also called myospasm.

Muscle spasm — tonic muscle spasm is a sustained involuntary muscle contraction resulting in pain and dysfunction.

Muscle spasticity — increased muscular tension of antagonists preventing normal movement and caused by an inability to relax (a loss of reciprocal inhibition).

Muscle tone — resting muscle activity. See also muscle hypertonicity.

Muscular atrophy — a wasting of muscular tissue, especially due to lack of use.

Muscular splinting — contraction of a muscle or group of muscles attended by interference with function and producing involuntary movement and distortion; differs from muscle spasm in that the contraction is not sustained when the muscle is at rest.

Musculoskeletal pain — deep, somatic pain that originates in skeletal muscles, fascial sheaths and tendons (myogenous pain), bone and periosteum (osseous pain), joint, joint capsules and ligaments (arthralgic pain), and soft connective tissues.

Mutually protected articulation — an occlusal scheme in which the posterior teeth prevent excessive contact of the anterior teeth in maximum intercuspation, and the anterior teeth disengage the posterior teeth in all mandibular excursive movements. Alternatively, an occlusal scheme in which the anterior teeth disengage the posterior teeth in all mandibular excursive movements, and the posterior teeth prevent excessive contact of the anterior teeth in maximum intercuspation.

Mutually protected occlusion — see mutually protected articulation.

Myalgia — pain in a muscle or muscles. See also facial arthromyalgia.

Myofascial pain and dysfunction — a syndrome that comprises, in various combinations – pain on palpation of the temporomandibular joint; pain on examination of the associated muscles; limitation or deviation of jaw movement; joint sounds; headache. Old term – pain dysfunction syndrome.

Myofascial trigger point — a hyperirritable spot, usually within a skeletal muscle or in the muscle fascia, that is painful on compression and can give rise to characteristic referred pain, tenderness (secondary hyperalgesia) and autonomic phenomena.

Myofunctional — relating to the function of muscles. In dentistry, the role of muscle function in the cause or correction of muscle-related problems.

Myofunctional therapy — the use of exercises to improve the action of a group of muscles used as an adjunct to orthodontic or craniomandibular dysfunction treatment.

Myogenous pain — deep somatic musculoskeletal pain originating in skeletal muscles, fascial sheaths or tendons.

Myositis — inflammation of muscle tissue.

Myospasm — see muscle spasm.

Myostatic contracture — muscle contracture resulting from reduced muscle stimulation.

Myotonia — increased muscular irritability and contractility with decreased power of relaxation; tonic muscle spasms.

Neck of the condylar process — the constricted inferior portion of the mandibular condylar process that is continuous with the ramus of the mandible; that portion of the condylar process that connects the mandibular ramus to the condyle.

Neurogenous pain — pain that is generated within the nervous system as a result of some abnormality of neural structures.

Neuromuscular dysfunction — a collective term for muscle disorders of the masticatory system with two observable major symptoms – pain and dysfunction. Common observations include muscle fatigue, muscle tightness, myalgia, spasm, headaches, decreased range of motion and acute malocclusion. The five types of masticatory muscle disorders include protective co-contraction (muscle splinting), local muscle soreness (non-inflammatory myalgia), myofascial pain (trigger point myalgia), myospasm (tonic contraction myalgia), and chronic centrally mediated myalgia (chronic myositis).

Neuromuscular release — a term used by some clinicians to describe a reduction in contractile and electric activity of the masticatory muscles.

Neuropathy — a general term used to designate an abnormality or pathological change in a peripheral nerve.

Non-steroidal anti-inflammatory drugs (NSAIDs) — a drug that has long-lasting analgesic and anti-inflammatory effects.

Non-working side — the side *from* which the mandible moves during lateral excursion.

Non-working side condyle path — the path that the condyle traverses on the non-working side when the mandible moves in a lateral excursion, which may be viewed in the three reference planes of the body.

Non-working side interference — a posterior occlusal contact on the non-working side, during lateral excursion of the mandible. See also non-working side.

Noxious stimulus — a tissue-damaging stimulus.

Occlude — to bring together; to shut; to bring or close the mandibular teeth into contact with the maxillary teeth.

Occlusal — pertaining to the masticatory surfaces of the posterior teeth, prostheses or occlusion rims.

Occlusal adjustment — any change in the occlusion intended to alter the occluding relation; any alteration of the occluding surfaces of the teeth or restorations.

Occlusal contact — the touching of opposing teeth on elevation of the mandible – any contact relation of opposing teeth. See also deflective occlusal contact; initial occlusal contact.

Occlusal disharmony — a phenomenon in which contacts of opposing occlusal surfaces are not in harmony with other tooth contacts and/or the anatomical and physiological components of the craniomandibular complex.

Occlusal force — the result of muscular force applied to opposing teeth; the force created by the dynamic action of the muscles during the physiological act of mastication; the result of muscular activity applied to opposing teeth.

Occlusal harmony — a condition in centric and eccentric jaw relation in which there are no interceptive or deflective contacts of occluding surfaces.

Occlusal interference — any tooth contact that inhibits the remaining occluding surfaces from achieving stable and harmonious contacts.

Occlusal prematurity — any contact of opposing teeth that occurs before the planned intercuspation.

Occlusal reduction — the quantity (usually measured in millimetres) of tooth structure that is removed to establish adequate space for a restorative material between the occlusal aspect of the tooth preparation and the opposing dentition.

Occlusal registration — a method of physically recording the contacts between the teeth.

Occlusal splint — an intraoral appliance of variable design used in the management of a temporomandibular disorder or parafunction.

Occlusal stability — the equalisation of contacts that prevents tooth movement after closure.

Occlusal trauma — trauma to the periodontium from functional or parafunctional forces causing damage to the attachment apparatus of the periodontium by exceeding its adaptive and reparative capacities. It may be self-limiting or progressive.

Occlusal vertical dimension — the distance measured between two points when the occluding members are in contact.

Occlusal wear — loss of substance on opposing occlusal units or surfaces as the result of attrition or abrasion.

Occlusion — the act or process of closure or of being closed or shut off; the static relationship between the incising or masticating surfaces of the maxillary or mandibular teeth or tooth analogues.

Occlusion analysis — a systematic examination of the masticatory system with special consideration to the effect of tooth occlusion on the teeth and their related structures.

Occlusion record — a registration of opposing occluding surfaces made at any maxillomandibular relationship.

Open lock — see TMJ locking.

Oromandibular dysfunction — see myofascial pain and dysfunction.

Ostectomy — the excision of bone or a portion of a bone, usually by means of a saw or chisel, for the removal of a sequestrum, the correction of a deformity, or any other purpose.

Osteoarthrosis — chronic degeneration and destruction of the articular cartilage and/or fibrous connective tissue linings of the joint components and discs, leading to bony spurs, pain, stiffness, limitation of movement and changes in bone morphology. Advanced conditions may involve erosions and disc degeneration with crepitus.

Pain dysfunction syndrome — see myofascial pain and dysfunction.

Panoramic radiograph — a tomogram of the maxilla and mandible taken with a specialised machine designed to present a panoramic view of the full circumferential lengths of the maxilla and mandible on a single film – also called orthopantograph.

Panoramic radiography — a method of radiography by which a continuous radiograph of the maxillary and/or mandibular dental arches and their associated structures may be obtained.

Parafunction — a function carried out to an abnormal degree (e.g. clenching, tooth grinding) during the day or night and of which the person may be unaware.

Passive manipulation — a technique for finding the path of closure to centric relation. See also centric relation.

Pathogenic occlusion — an occlusal relationship capable of producing pathological changes in the stomatognathic system.

Physical elasticity of muscle — the physical quality of muscle of being elastic, i.e. yielding to active or passive physical stretch.

Physiological elasticity of muscle — the unique biological quality of muscle of being capable of change and of resuming its size under neuromuscular control.

Physiological occlusion — occlusion in harmony with the functions of the masticatory system.

Physiologically balanced occlusion — a balanced occlusion that is in harmony with the temporomandibular joints and the neuromuscular system.

Placebo effect — a physical or emotional effect not directly attributable to any specific property of a therapeutic agent.

Plain radiography — basic two-dimensional imaging using an X-ray source and conventional film/cassettes.

Polyvinylsiloxane — a silicone elastomeric impression material of silicone polymers that has terminal vinyl groups that cross-link with silanes on activation by a platinum or palladium salt catalyst.

Posterior band of the intra-articular disc — a component of the intra-articular disc interposed between the head of the condyle and the articular fossa, when the mandible is at rest.

Posterior bilaminar zone — the posterior part of the intra-articular disc comprising two parts – (a) elastic attachment to the articular fossa and (b) fibrous attachment to the neck of the condyle. See also elastic attachment; fibrous attachment.

Posterior guidance — guidance of the mandible during eccentric movements as provided by the temporomandibular joint. See also anterior guidance; ideal anterior guidance.

Posterior interference — any predominant contact between the back teeth on excentric movements of the mandible.

Premature contact in CR — first tooth contact when mandible is in centric relation.

Protrusion — movement of the mandible relative to the maxilla that is primarily in an anterior direction. See also lateral protrusion.

Protrusive — thrusting forward; adjective denoting protrusion.

Protrusive condyle path — the path that the condyle travels when the mandible is moved forward from its initial position.

Protrusive deflection — a continuing excentric displacement of the midline incisal path on protrusion, symptomatic of a restriction of movement.

Protrusive deviation — discursive movement on protrusion that ends in the centred position and is indicative of interference during movement.

Protrusive interocclusal record — a registration of the mandible in relation to the maxilla when both condyles are advanced in the temporal fossa.

Protrusive jaw relation — a jaw relation resulting from protrusion of the mandible.

Protrusive movement — mandibular movement anterior to centric relation.

Protrusive occlusion — an occlusion of the teeth when the mandible is protruded.

Protrusive record — see protrusive interocclusal record.

Protrusive relation — the relation of the mandible to the maxillae when the mandible is thrust forward.

Psychogenic facial pain — facial pain not associated with organic disease which may have a psychosomatic aetiology.

Pterygoid plates — broad, thin, wing-shaped processes of the sphenoid bone separated by the pterygoid fossa. The inferior end of the medial plate terminates in a long curved process or hook for the tendon of the tensor veli palatini muscle. The lateral plate gives attachment to the medial and lateral pterygoid muscles.

Rad — acronym for radiation absorbed dose, a unit of measurement of the absorbed dose of ionising radiation. The biological effect of 1 rad varies with the type of radiation to which tissue is exposed.

Range of motion — the range, measured in degrees of a circle, through which a joint can be extended or flexed. The range of the opening, lateral, and protrusive excursions of the temporomandibular joint.

Reciprocal click — clicks emanating from the temporomandibular joint, one of which occurs during opening movement and the other during closing movement.

Registration — the making of a record of the jaw relationships present, or those desired, thus allowing their transfer to an articulator to assist in proper fabrication of a dental prosthesis – a record made of the desired maxillomandibular relationship and used to relate casts to an articulator.

REM period of sleep (rapid eye movement) — an active period of sleep usually just before waking, during which there are periods of increased muscle activity.

Remodel — the morphological change in bone as an adaptive response to altered environmental demands. The bone will progressively remodel where there is a proliferation of tissue and regressive remodelling when osteoclastic resorption is evident.

Resisted movement test — a technique of muscle examination by inducing forced contraction usually employed in examining the lateral pterygoid muscle.

Retrodiscal tissue — see bilaminar zone.

Retruded contact — contact of a tooth or teeth along the retruded path of closure. Initial contact of a tooth or teeth during closure around a transverse horizontal axis.

Retruded contact position (RCP) — a synonym for centric relation.

Scintigraphy — a method of imaging in which patients are injected with a radiopharmaceutical. The pharmaceutical component locates to the cells or tissues of interest while the radioactive component emits gamma rays that can be detected using a gamma camera.

Semi-adjustable articulator — an articulator that permits replication of average mandibular movements.

Shimstock — a thin (8–12 µm) strip of polyester film used to identify the presence or absence of occlusal or proximal contacts.

Short-wave diathermy — electrophysiotherapy with a primarily thermal effect, causing increased blood flow.

Soft bite guard (soft splint) — resilient polyvinyl vacuum formed device covering either the mandibular teeth made to no particular occlusion for the suggested purpose of preventing trauma to the dentition.

Somatisation — the expression of personal and social distress in an idiom of physical bodily complaints with medical help seeking.

Sphenomandibular ligament — a ligament running from the sphenoid process to the lingula on the mesial aspect of the mandible.

Splint — see occlusal splint.

Stabilisation splint — a hard acrylic splint designed to provide an ideal occlusion. Synonyms – Michigan splint, Tanner appliance, Fox appliance, centric relation appliance.

Static occlusion — the contacts between the teeth when the mandible is closed in centric occlusion.

Stomatognathic system — the combination of structures involved in speech, receiving, mastication and deglutition as well as parafunctional actions.

Study cast — see diagnostic cast.

Stylomandibular ligament — a ligament running from the styloid process to the posterior border of the mandible at the angle. May become calcified later in life.

Subluxation — an incomplete or partial dislocation that is self-reducing. See also Condylar subluxation.

Superior pterygoid — the superior head of the lateral pterygoid muscle inserted into the anterior extension of the intra-articular disc. Active in the close/ clench cycle. See also lateral pterygoid.

Synovial fluid — a viscid fluid contained in joint cavities and secreted by the synovial membrane.

Synovial membrane — the articular membrane composed of specialised endothelial cells capable of producing synovial fluid, filling the joint cavity surrounded by the membrane.

Tanner appliance — see stabilisation splint.

Temporalis muscle — a muscle originating from the temporal fossa, running below the zygomatic arch to insert into the anterior aspect of the coronoid process. In normal function, one of the principal elevator muscles.

Temporomandibular disorders (TMDs) — a collective term encompassing conditions that affect the articulatory system.

Temporomandibular joint (TMJ) — the articulation of the condylar process of the mandible and the intra-articular disc with the mandibular fossa of the squamous portion of the temporal bone; a diarthrodial sliding and rotating joint. Movement in the upper joint compartment is mostly translational, whereas that in the lower joint compartment is mostly rotational. The joint connects the mandibular condyle to the articular fossa of the temporal bone with the temporomandibular disc interposed.

Temporomandibular joint hypermobility — excessive mobility of the temporomandibular joint

Temporomandibular ligament — see lateral ligament.

TENS — acronym for transcutaneous electrical neural stimulation

Tension-type headache — may be episodic or chronic. The headache is usually pressing or tightening in quality, of mild or moderate intensity, bilateral and does not worsen with physical activity. The term 'tension' is related to muscle contraction not psychological stress.

Terminal hinge axis — the axis of closure when the mandible is in centric relation. See also Centric relation.

TMJ locking — a restricted mandibular movement due to a mechanical cause, usually associated with disc displacement; may be open or closed.

Tomogram — a radiograph made by using a tomograph.

Tomograph — a device for moving an X-ray source in one direction as the film moves in the opposite direction; a radiograph produced from a machine that has the source of radiation moving in one direction and the film moving in the opposite direction.

Tomography — a general term for a technique that provides a distinct image of any selected plane through the body, while the images of structures that lie above and below that plane are blurred. Also, the term body-section radiography has been applied to the procedure, although the several ways of accomplishing it have been given distinguishing names.

Tongue habit — conscious or unconscious movements of the tongue that are not related to purposeful functions. Such habits may produce malocclusion or injuries to tissues of the tongue or the attachment apparatus of the teeth.

Tongue scalloping — scalloping of the tongue with characteristic indentations along the lateral border of the tongue; taken as a sign of active bruxism.

Tongue thrusting — the infantile pattern of suckle–swallow in which the tongue is placed between the incisor teeth or alveolar ridges during the initial stages of deglutition, resulting sometimes in an anterior open occlusion, deformation of the jaws, and/or abnormal function.

Transcranial oblique radiograph — a radiographic projection in which the central beam travels across the cranium at a 20° angle through the skull from the opposite side, showing an oblique lateral view of the condyle and fossa.

Transcutaneous electrical neural stimulation (TENS) — application of low-voltage electrical stimulation through the skin to nerves in order to interfere with the sensation of pain in the brain and increase blood flow to the region. A method of physiotherapy used in the treatment of musculoskeletal disorders.

Transient mandibular deviation — a mandibular pathway where there is a deviation to one side and then back to the midline at maximum opening. This could imply that there is a temporary obstruction to smooth mandibular movement, possibly due to disc displacement with reduction.

Translation — that motion of a rigid body in which a straight line passing through any two points always remains parallel to its initial position. The motion may be described as a sliding or gliding motion.

Translatory movement — the motion of a body at any instant when all points within the body are moving at the same velocity and in the same direction.

Transpharyngeal radiograph — this is a plain radiograph taken with the mouth open and the centre beam directed through the contralateral sigmoid notch to show bony detail of the neck and head of the condyle.

Tricyclic antidepressants — a group of antidepressant drugs that, when administered in low doses, have mild analgesic and muscle relaxant properties, independent of their anxiolytic effect.

Trigger point — irritable focus in a soft-tissue structure, most commonly muscle, which, when stimulated, is locally tender and may give rise to referred pain.

Trismus — a reduced ability to open the mouth, due to increased tonic contraction of muscle.

Ultrasound — electrophysiotherapy employing sound waves to produce thermal and mechanical effects in the tissue.

Unstrained jaw relation — the relation of the mandible to the skull when a state of balanced tonus exists among all the muscles involved; any jaw relation that is attained without undue or unnatural force and that causes no undue distortion of the tissues of the temporomandibular joints.

Vascular headache — a headache associated with a vascular disorder in which the onset, or worsening, of a pre-existing headache disorder is in close time relation to the vascular disorder.

Vertical axis of the mandible — an imaginary line around which the mandible may rotate through the horizontal plane.

Vertical dimension — the distance between two selected anatomical or marked points (usually one on the tip of the nose and the other on the chin), one on a fixed and one on a movable member.

Vertical dimension decrease — decreasing the vertical distance between the mandible and the maxillae by modifications of teeth, the positions of teeth or occlusion rims, or through alveolar or residual ridge resorption.

Vertical dimension increase — increasing the vertical distance between the mandible and the maxillae by modifications of teeth, the positions of teeth or occlusion rims.

Wear facets — see facet.

Whiplash — the characteristic head and neck motion that occurs when a relatively rigid thorax is suddenly accelerated or decelerated independently of the head. It describes a hyper-extension/flexion injury to the soft tissues of the neck.

Working side — the side *to which* the mandible moves during lateral excursion.

Working side condyle — the condyle on the working side.

Working side condyle path — the path that the condyle travels on the working side when the mandible moves in a lateral excursion.

Working side contacts — contacts of teeth made on the side of the articulation towards which the mandible is moved during working movements.

Working side interference — a posterior occlusal contact on the working side, during lateral excursion of the mandible. See also working side.

Further Reading

Academy of Prosthodontics (2017). The glossary of prosthodontic terms. *J Prosthet Dent* 55: e1–e105.

Gray, R.J.M., Davies, S., and Quayle, A.A. (1997). A clinical guide to temporomandibular disorders. *Br Dent J* 177: 135–142.

Gray, R. and Al-Ani, Z. (2010). Risk management in clinical practice. Part 8. Temporomandibular disorders. *Br Dent J* 209: 433–449.

Appendix III

Short Answer Questions

Please see www.wiley.com/go/al-ani/temporomandibular-disorders-2e for multiple-choice questions related to this book.

1. Disc morphology: the intra-articular disc as being like a 'school-boy's cap'. It is an oval-shaped tense sheet of fibrous tissue with a concave inferior surface sitting on the head of the condyle. Label the structures on the following image.

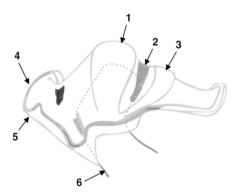

2. Signs and symptoms of temporomandibular disorders (TMDs) are more common in females. Discuss.
3. The lower limit of normal movement in millimetres is:
4. Female: Vertical   _____   Lateral   _____
5. Male: Vertical   _____   Lateral   _____

6. What might vary the ranges of movement and how?
7. What causes a click?

Temporomandibular Disorders: A Problem-Based Approach, Second Edition. M. Ziad Al-Ani and Robin J.M. Gray.
© 2021 M. Ziad Al-Ani and Robin J.M. Gray. Published 2021 by John Wiley & Sons Ltd.
Companion Website: www.wiley.com/go/al-ani/temporomandibular-disorders-2e

8. How do you examine the lateral pterygoid muscle? Can you justify its intra-oral examination?
9. What does crepitus indicate?
10. Are TMD symptoms common in F/F denture wearers?
11. Based on your understanding of the anatomy knowledge, what is the most reliable method of palpating the temporomandibular joint (TMJ)?
12. Is there one splint of choice in the treatment of TMD?
13. Do drugs have a place in the management of TMD? If so, what drugs and when?
14. Should headache be treated by dentists?
15. What is the most common TMD?
16. What are the signs of active bruxism?
17. What are the medicolegal aspects of patient care that we should always bear in mind?
18. Is there an important psychological aspect of TMD that we should consider?
19. Are radiographs important in the consideration of the management of TMD and the development of a treatment plan?
20. What provides the posterior guidance of the mandible? Explain your answer?
21. What provides the anterior guidance of the mandible? Explain your answer?
22. What are the classic symptoms of myofascial pain?
23. What are the classic symptoms of osteoarthrosis?
24. What is meant by the term second-phase TMD treatment? Is this recommended, if so/not why?
25. Is occlusal adjustment justified as a first-line treatment option? Is this recommended, if so/not why?
26. Should occlusal appliances be full coverage? If not, why?
27. At what time of the day should splints be worn? Give reasons?
28. Are occlusal interferences a cause or a result of a TMD?
29. Does orthodontic treatment cause TMD?
30. Is there enough evidence to use botulinum toxin injections for bruxism management?

Index